The Nursing Home Handbook

A Guide for Families

The Nursing Home Handbook

A Guide for Families

Jo Horne

An AARP Book
published by
American Association of Retired Persons
Washington, D.C.

Scott, Foresman and Company
Glenview, Illinois

Library of Congress Cataloging-in-Publication Data

Horne, Jo.
  The nursing home handbook.

  Bibliography: p.
  Includes index.
  1. Nursing homes—Handbooks, manuals, etc. I. Title.
CDNLM: 1. Homes for the Aged—United States. 2. Long
Term Care. 3. Nursing Homes—United States.
WT 27 AA1 H8n]
RA997.H675 1989   362.1′6′0973   89-6007

1 2 3 4 5 6 RRC 94 93 92 91 90 89

To Larry—
whose respect for older people got me into this
business of writing in the first place
whose knowledge and ability to edit
made him almost a coauthor
and whose constant strength and belief
in me make everything possible.

Acknowledgments

With special appreciation to . . .

Katie Aker, Donna Ambrogi, Michael Bredeck, Jackie Ceilie, Mary Deshler, Anne Dowling, Shirley Ellis, Jane Engbring, Cathy Gerdes, Laurie Hackett, Joanne Hiller, Maggie Janz, Kathy Kliman, Luetta Koepke, Irene Long, Karen McKenna, Johnel Moore, Tim Ressel, Lisa Schini, Dorothy Wright, and the twenty-eight ombudspersons who took the time and energy to respond to a comprehensive survey.

The author also gratefully acknowledges the support of the Midwest Geriatric Education Center of Marquette University. Without the input of the staff and faculty, this project would not have been nearly as rewarding as it has been.

Preface

I began thinking about writing this book three years ago following the publication of *Caregiving: Helping an Aging Loved One*, a handbook for those giving care to family members in the community. There seemed to be a clear need for hands-on information for caregivers faced with the nursing home dilemma. Researching the available resources, I discovered that while there was a great deal of information (mostly in the form of booklets and handouts) to help in the actual selection process when choosing a home, there was little about how the decision is made in the first place. And discussion of what the family role becomes once a person moves into a nursing home was practically nonexistent.

The clear need was for a handbook that did not end with the older person being moved into his or her room in the nursing home. The development of this handbook in answer to that need followed a path of information seeking, interviews, and visits around the country. Every state ombudsperson program was contacted for input, and twenty-eight programs responded. Interviews were willingly given by family members who had made the decision in favor of a nursing home, family members who had chosen an alternative, nursing home residents, frail older persons not living in nursing homes, ombudspersons, hospital discharge planners, nursing home administrators, activity and social services personnel, and other professionals in the field of geriatrics.

Having recently completed a book on housing alternatives for older persons both able and frail, I was interested to see what life in a nursing home could offer that one of the alternatives could not fulfill. In researching homes, I took on the persona of a daughter looking into the possibility of nursing home care for one of her frail parents who might move to the city from out of state. I also visited homes in rural areas presenting myself as the daughter of persons living in that area. Sometimes I visited homes as the author of this handbook. None of the scenarios was a lie, and each yielded interesting and unique perspectives for the project.

In my years of work as a writer on aging, a director of an adult daycare center, and a speaker and consultant, I have found the prevailing attitude toward nursing homes to be one of *never:* "I will *never* go there" or "I will *never* allow my parent (or spouse) to go there." But in those same years, I have come to appreciate the need for the nursing home as a vital component of the long-term care program offered in the United States. My hope for the reader is that after reading this handbook, he or she will come to the same conclusion.

Nursing homes are here to stay. Beyond helping the caregiving family to come to a decision and select an appropriate home for a loved one, my aim is to inspire caregivers to become interested enough in the nursing home industry as a whole to take an active role in bringing it more fully into the growing list of acceptable long-term care options.

Contents

PART TWO

Chapter 8: MAKING THE ADJUSTMENT

P·A·R·T
ONE

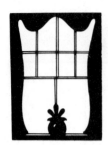

Chapter 1

A Caregiver's Toughest Decision

Nursing home. Traditionally, these words strike fear or, at the very least, dread in the hearts of older persons and their family members and friends. And yet for 1.5 million Americans, these words describe the place they live. The most often quoted sources report that only 5 percent of the population reside in nursing homes, but also that one in five or 20 percent of all Americans will spend some time in nursing homes during their lives. It is encouraging to note that for every person who lives in a nursing home, two persons with the same degree of impairment are living in the community. Institutionalization is never a foregone conclusion just because someone is old and frail, but when it is an answer, caregivers can take some comfort from the fact that there are good nursing homes in the United States. This book is designed to help you find one.

When Placement Is Indicated

To the uninitiated, a nursing home may be the choice of last resort, a place where old and infirm persons are confined by their relatives to spend their last days. This is certainly not the case. Many people live in nursing homes by their own choice. And in many cases, a nursing home stay will be short-term rather than permanent. In today's streamlined world of health care, it is not uncommon for a hospital to provide care until the patient is stabilized and then transfer that patient to a nursing home for the kind of rehabilitative and convalescent care once provided as part of a hospitalization. Nursing homes, therefore, can be considered as just one aspect in the process of providing long-term care to older people.

So when the physician or social worker says "nursing home," do not think the worst. What these health care professionals may be suggesting is a continuation of care that can be better provided in the setting of a nursing and rehabilitative facility.

Sometimes, of course, a permanent change in residence is needed. These days, persons who are taking up permanent residence in nursing homes are in general older, sicker, and more frail than such residents were in the past. The important message here is that the community is able to provide services which allow older persons to stay independent and be cared for outside of an institution for a much longer period of time.

You need to understand this change in the type of person who resides in nursing homes today, because when you tour nursing homes in the process of selecting a place for your relative, you may be shocked at the level of frailty and illness you see there. People who have never spent any time visiting or volunteering in nursing homes are frequently overwhelmed when they first walk into a home. Their first impressions are of very old people who are noticeably sick, feeble, and incapacitated. This can be a frightening and unnerving experience if one is not prepared.

Basically, there are four situations under which most placements are made:

- the emergency placement directly from the hospital
- the emergency placement from the home
- the planned placement arranged for the person by his or her family or caregivers
- the planned placement arranged for by the individual older person

The Emergency Placement
Many of you who are caregivers will find that the emergency placement develops out of an acute crisis. In this case, the need for nursing home care will come suddenly and

perhaps even shockingly. Your search for a suitable home will need to be conducted under stress and with haste. You had thought you would be able to take Dad home again following his latest stroke, but you are told that he needs more care than you can possibly give at home, that he "belongs" in a nursing home, and that you may have as little as forty-eight hours to find one.

It is possible that this placement directly from the hospital may be for purposes of rehabilitation and convalescence and that if all goes well, your relative will be able to return home after a short-term residency in the nursing home. Or the need may have come following a series of hospitalizations where each time the need for care has escalated until now the professionals insist the best choice is care in a nursing home. In either case, the task is to find the best available home.

In either case, you have some real help available to you. In many communities there are professionals called *case managers*. These individuals are trained to assist clients and their families in managing the details of a long-term care plan. Case managers are employed by both public and private agencies. The social services staff and discharge planners employed by the hospital also know the process, and they know what is available in your community. They can do a lot of the ground work for you, and that is important because, as you will learn, in this situation you are often going to be under pressure to make a choice in a very limited amount of time.

Have you heard someone mention a DRG? This acronym stands for *diagnostic-related groups*, and it affects people on Medicare in hospitals by controlling the number of days a person can stay in the hospital for any particular illness or condition.

This labeling and grouping of illnesses according to "normal" hospital stays often intensifies the process of finding a nursing home for a hospitalized patient. You need to understand that for the most part, the physician and social services staff have little control over these rules. One hospital discharge planner reported with a heavy sigh, "By the time we get the order to go looking for the nursing home, the chances are the hospital already has allocated the hospital bed for another patient."

If the placement will take place from the hospital, social services staff and discharge planners may offer the following assistance:

• They will sit in on the meeting where the doctor tells the patient he or she needs nursing home care.

• They will follow up with some counseling for both the patient and the family.

• They will offer some explanation and information on determining pay source (how the nursing home will be paid for).

• They will call some homes and ask those homes to evaluate the patient to determine whether the home can meet the patient's needs.

• They will recommend several homes for the family to tour, doing the prescreening work (see pages 45–49) for the family.

• If Title XIX (Medicaid) is to be the pay source, they will make the appointment for screening for Medicaid.

• They will facilitate the paperwork and arrange for transportation to the home on the day of discharge.

• They will answer questions, and when they do not have answers, they will suggest a resource for getting the answer.

• Once the move has taken place, they will remain available for a brief period of time for the family to speak with in the event of further questions or problems.

The hospital discharge planner and/or social worker CANNOT:

• make the final choice of the home (having the hospital staff choose the home is not a way to take away your guilt)

• give specific financial or legal advice

• extend indefinitely the time the patient and family can have to find a nursing home

• guarantee the patient will get the nursing home of first choice.

If you have been giving care at home, you may find yourself in a crisis situation that convinces you to make an immediate change in the care arrangements. Perhaps you have been caring for your wife, who has Alzheimer's disease. Things have gone from bad to worse: She no longer recognizes you; she constantly tries to leave the house; she has become a danger to herself. You cannot watch her twenty-four hours a day. Something must be done and quickly.

Or you live several hundred miles away from your mother. She lives in a remote rural area where services are limited. You have been concerned for some time about her ability to manage the aging and secluded house. She has a history of health problems that have resulted in multiple hospitalizations plus medications over the last several years. You get a call from a concerned neighbor who tells you she found your mother unconscious yesterday. When you talk to the doctor, he advises you that your mother is endangering herself by continuing to live alone in such isolated circumstances. He tells you her unconsciousness came about because she had been improperly medicating herself with prescribed and over-the-counter drugs.

These are but two examples of situations where a nursing home may be an option, again for either short-term or permanent residency. If you are trying to deal with an emergency placement while the person is still living at home, you can also get professional help.

When there is no hospital or agency involved to help you and you are under pressure to choose in a hurry:

- Begin with the person's physician and seek his or her advice on what to do.
- Rely on the assistance of any community agencies your relative may be receiving services from.
- Call the local Office on Aging for advice on how to proceed.
- Call some nursing homes and ask to speak with the admissions counselor.

- Call the local ombudsperson—this is a state-appointed (but federally mandated) advocate for residents of nursing homes and their families.
- Follow the steps outlined in the coming chapters.

Whether the emergency placement is from the hospital or from home, do yourself (and your relative) a favor and use the professionals available to you. They bring two very important ingredients to the process: experience and objectivity.

The Planned Placement

Others of you may be in the position of having more time to make a choice. You have been giving care and the situation has worsened. The person is living alone in another community. The care needs have grown. If you are the on-site caregiver, perhaps you are tired and overcommitted. Your own health is being jeopardized. Your spouse or children need more attention. Your work needs more attention.

Some of you may need to consider a nursing home because a change in the person's condition makes it impossible for you to continue to give care at home. For example, if the person has Parkinson's disease and gradually becomes less and less ambulatory, you may be unable to handle the sheer physical work of helping this person move from place to place.

If you have thought that a nursing home might become a reality at some point in the future, you can start now to collect some data and facts that will make the selection process easier.

Finally, in a few cases the older person decides that a nursing home is the right choice. This person has taken stock of his or her situation and decided that residency in a nursing home would be a positive move. As the caregiver, you can help this person by assisting him or her in collecting data, touring and evaluating homes, and managing the details of the actual move.

How to Use This Book

This book has been written as a handbook for those caregivers who are considering or may, at some future time, consider the possibility of a nursing home as a care center for their relatives. Why address the caregiver and not the person moving to the nursing home? Because statistically you will most likely be the one to choose and to decide. At the time the decision is made, the older person may be too sick and/or disoriented to have much input. If your relative is competent, however, you need to make every effort to include him or her in these momentous decisions that will affect his or her lifestyle.

You will be able to use the following pages to take you and your relative (and the rest of the family) step by step through the usually stressful process of choosing a home, helping the person move and adjust, and monitoring the care and quality of life once the person resides there.

Whether you are choosing a nursing home in a hurry or have plenty of time to consider all possibilities, the basic process is the same:

1. Assess the needs and talk to the patient.
2. Understand and choose the best payment sources for the care needed.
3. Prescreen possible nursing homes.
4. Tour the most likely nursing homes.
5. Check the state survey records for those homes that seem most promising.
6. Discuss the most likely homes with the patient.
7. Take a second look at the most likely homes.
8. Prepare for moving day with the older person.

These are the steps in *choosing* a nursing home. Following the actual move, the caregiver needs to continue to offer support and concern as the older person adjusts to the new residence and the sometimes radical changes in lifestyle.

The point to keep in mind is that the only difference in the selection process for a caregiver in a hurry and for one who plans for the possibility well in advance of the event is *time*.

What You Need to Understand before Beginning

You need to know a few basic rules regardless of whether the search for a nursing home comes about as a result of an emergency or as part of a planned process to continue care at the highest possible level.

1. Anyone can apply to any nursing home in any state regardless of residency in that state.
2. Many nursing homes are filled to capacity and have long waiting lists.
3. Nursing homes have to be Medicare and/or Medicaid *certified* in order to be eligible to receive those funds.
4. There are stringent financial rules and strict guidelines for application to receive Title XIX (Medicaid) assistance.
5. While they vary from state to state, laws that govern practically every aspect of design, decor, management, and operation of nursing homes are backed up by annual inspections.
6. A potential resident may be turned away for any number of reasons including lack of bed, lack of sufficient staff, level of care needed, type of plan for payment, mental illness, and disruptive or abusive behavior.
7. While a high level of care may be given, a nursing home is not a hospital. You will not see constant interaction between the nursing staff and the residents. On the other hand, a nursing home is not a rest home or hotel. You should see solid evidence that care is being given and is available when called for.

As you go through the process, you will learn about the place of the nursing home in our society and how that place differs dramatically from what it was just ten years ago. Issues about quality of care and regulations for achieving that care are being debated even as this book goes to press. There are major changes in the making; there are major changes already on the books that are going to affect the kind of lifestyle your relative may have in a nursing home. Two key pieces of federal legislation are already having an impact on the nursing home industry. The Omnibus Budget Reconciliation Act of 1987 includes the first major federal reforms for regulating quality of care in nursing homes to be enacted since the passage of Medicare. And the Medicare Catastrophic Coverage Act of 1988 includes an important provision to protect couples against spousal impoverishment if one partner needs nursing home care. (See page 34.)

Today's nursing home is very different from the nursing homes of just a few years ago. Today, residents more frequently come into the home later in life, and they are more frail and ill than ever before. Many residents need high-level care—care that a few years ago would have been offered only in the hospital. Nursing home personnel are constantly having to learn new nursing skills or update old ones. And while a few years ago nursing homes may have seemed like retirement or rest homes where the greatest need was custodial care, today more and more homes are working with residents who need continuous nursing care.

No single nursing home is going to meet all your criteria for caring for your relative. And no nursing home—regardless of how good it is—can possibly provide the kind of one-to-one personal care and attention you give at home. Nursing homes are run by mortal men and women as prone to mistakes as anyone else. You are going to have some serious emotions with which to deal. While attitudes are changing toward older people in our society, the fact remains that nursing homes are still looked upon as an absolute last resort. The very language used to describe residency there is negative: "nursing home *placement*," "*putting* Mom in a nursing home," "the need to *institutionalize*," "Dad is *in a home*" (as opposed to "Dad lives at the Manor").

In some cases, nursing homes may attempt to disguise their real functions as institutions. Many nursing homes will suggest to families who tour that the home is a "convalescent center" or "rehabilitation center" or even "rest or retirement home." But your relative is not simple-minded—even if there is mental impairment. He or she knows what a nursing home looks like. He or she has some ideas (whether right or wrong) about what residency there can mean. He or she should not be insulted by euphemisms.

As you move through this difficult process, do yourself and your relative a favor. Be as direct and honest as the situation allows you to be, both with yourself and your relative. It will not all go smoothly. There are going to be moments when you wonder about the rightness of this decision. There are going to be pressures—subtle and overt— from all sides. But do not concern yourself with satisfying the expectations and dogmas of either society or other family and friends. Your purpose in this process is threefold:

1. to ascertain if the nursing home is the best (or only) answer for your relative and you
2. to find the very best home for and, if possible, with your relative
3. to assume your revised caregiving role as advocate for your relative and as teammate with the staff of the home

You are not going to do a perfect job of this. In spite of the work you do gathering all the information, making all the notes, and going back for a second visit, the bottom line still may be choosing a place that is several notches below what you had hoped for. But once you help the person move, there are ways in which you and your relative can make the best of even a less-than-perfect living situation.

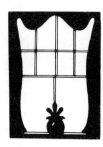

Chapter 2

Assessing the Situation

When is it time to consider the possibility of nursing home care?

This can be a tough question. On the one hand, you do not want to consider nursing home placement until you have exhausted every other means of maintaining the older person in the community as independently and autonomously as possible. Caregivers need to understand that when some new issue of care arises, it is not necessarily time to push the panic button and go looking for a nursing home.

On the other hand, the wise caregiver begins to think about and prepare for the possibility as far in advance as is reasonable.

Paradox? Not really. Consider this case:

Laura is living with her daughter. She attends a daycare center every day while her daughter works. She uses a wheelchair to get around since her stroke and needs help with dressing, bathing, and toileting. She is diabetic and has had two recent hospitalizations with complications brought on by the diabetes.

This situation warrants some initial research into the idea that a nursing home may become a necessity at some time in the near future.

One more case:

Roland has been diagnosed as having Alzheimer's disease. His condition has been manageable for several years, and he has remained at home under the care of his wife, Marie. But recently he has been up several times at night and has sometimes not recognized his wife or his home. Marie is beginning to experience some health problems of her own—problems her doctor warns her are worsened by the continuous stress and demands of her caregiving.

Marie certainly needs to begin to make some plans. She may find other ways to have Roland stay at home or in the community, but the time has come (and perhaps is well past) for her to take some action. Given the prognosis of Alzheimer's, even if she does find some stopgap measures for now, the chances are that she may need to consider a nursing home at some time before the illness runs its course.

Are Nursing Homes Really Necessary?

In many cases, the nursing home is still viewed as a retirement center, and, as was noted earlier, many first-time visitors are shocked at the level of care needed by and given to today's nursing home resident.

"I was perfectly ignorant about the whole thing," reported one seventy-eight-year-old caregiver about to seek a home for her husband. "I never even considered the idea of a nursing home either for myself or my husband."

Such reactions are hardly uncommon. Misconceptions about nursing homes abound. Nursing home scandal makes such juicy and shocking reading that people—especially older people—may have the idea that all nursing homes are bad and evil places. Another misconception is that a facility will be very similar to a hospital.

The truth is that the nursing home is an important component in the continuum of care available for older Americans. The nursing home plays a valuable role in its ability to offer care and safe haven to those whose needs can no longer be adequately met elsewhere in the community.

Keeping someone in clear need out of a nursing home because of a misplaced sense of duty or pride or because you promised "never" can be detrimental not only to that person's mental and physical well-being but to your own. Your role is to assist your relative in making a careful choice and then to monitor the care provided for any signs of problems.

There will be pluses and minuses in any nursing home residency. Potentially the most serious problems are that adequate care will not be provided and that the person will be abused. Caregivers are also concerned about the possibility of infection, serious falls, worsening of incontinence and confusion, and lessening of mobility.

Potential problems also include the social impacts of moving into a nursing home. Relocation is traumatic at any age; relocation for an older person can be catastrophic. Emotions that must be dealt with include the loss of control, the feeling of dependence and helplessness, the feeling of worthlessness, and depersonalization. There are also other realities to be faced such as loss of financial security and control, loss of role in community, loss of social supports and networks, plus having to deal with the frequent sensory overload of this new environment. In Part Two of this book, you will learn ways to help reduce the stress of relocation.

Considering all these potential problems, who on earth would choose nursing home care either for themselves or for someone they love? Believe it or not, some of those same negatives can be positives. It is true that people die in nursing homes. It is also true that people die in hospitals and at home. Most people who live in nursing homes are at the ends of their lives. The nursing home does not precipitate death. Death in a nursing home may follow a long illness and may come to the person as he or she is surrounded by caring family and professionals who are there to make death as painless as possible.

While circumstances exist for infection and falls, caregivers also need to consider the fact that nursing homes are designed specifically for frail older people and are equipped with handrails, grab bars, and emergency call bells as well as safety and security measures the resident probably does not have elsewhere in the community. A fall at home may have brought about the need for nursing home care in the first place. Residents also have easier access to care and attention, therapy, and care plans that regulate such details. Nutrition and medication are carefully monitored, and families often find that a relative gets better care in these areas from the nursing home because at home he or she was not eating properly and frequently mixed up medications.

Socially, many nursing home residents actually thrive once they become acclimated to the new environment. Long deprived of social contact in many cases, they enjoy the comings and goings and interactions with staff and other residents. At some levels of care, residents are able to enjoy not only opportunities to make friends and try activities, but possibilities for self-expression and self-actualization as well. And while many caregivers fret and worry over the action of "putting" their relatives in nursing homes, many family members are surprised to discover that over time their relationship with the person actually is enriched once the burden of constant care is handled by someone outside the family.

How do you go about finding the best possible home? Set some basic standards before you begin to look. It is not enough for a home to be clean and beautifully decorated. It is not enough for the staff to be friendly. For your relative, you want more. You seek intangibles that will lie beneath the facade including:

- recognition of each resident as an individual
- focus on possibility rather than disability
- focus on independence rather than dependence
- recognition of residents, staff, and caregivers as a team
- emphasis on "humanizing" the environment
- emphasis on quality care supported by employee training and incentive programs
- recognition of role of the nursing home as a part of the total community

What Are the Indicators for Placement?

What markers and guides are available for caregivers to ascertain the possibility a nursing home might be needed at some point?

Age is one. For persons over sixty-five, the possibility for institutionalization increases with each decade of life.

Persons who live alone may be at higher risk than those who live with someone else—even if that other person also has impairments.

Health naturally plays a role. Most older persons have at least one chronic condition—arthritis, diabetes, heart disease, or hearing or visual impairment, to name a few. Many older people have several chronic conditions. Chronic illness has a number of common denominators: The course of the illness is uncertain—it can escalate unexpectedly into an acute situation; the condition often involves pain, discomfort, disability, and most certainly some restrictions on levels of activity; the condition intrudes into the lives of not only the patient but the caregiver; and the condition sometimes requires the use of a number of outside services such as delivery of meals, transportation services, and in-home help and care. When a chronic situation ignites into an acute or catastrophic event, that change in health status may mean a need for a higher level of care—at least for a while.

Another indicator may be *personal care activities*. Persons who have difficulty and need help with one or more activities of personal care such as bathing, dressing, eating, transferring from chair to bed, walking, getting out of the house, or managing personal hygiene (toileting themselves) are at a higher risk for institutionalization.

The *ability to manage* the basic activities of daily living in a home also enters the picture. If a person needs help shopping, preparing meals, managing money, using the telephone, and/or maintaining the home, he or she may possibly be in the high risk category.

How Do You Assess Needs?

In the emergency placement situation, someone from the nursing home may visit your relative either in the hospital or at home for the purpose of determining care needs. One of the issues this assessment will determine is whether or not that particular nursing home has space in the appropriate unit to care for your relative.

This may also be the stage where the patient finds out nursing home care is being proposed. (See pages 25–28.) The hospital staff will handle the assessment. Your part begins when it is time to tell the person he or she needs nursing home care. Plan to be with the patient for this. Let the physician, hospital social worker, and/or discharge planner deliver the news that a stay in a nursing home is to be prescribed, but be present during this conversation so that there is no opportunity for misunderstanding.

Ask questions. Seek information both for yourself and for the patient. Talk privately with your relative once the professionals have left. Acknowledge that the news is difficult and perhaps even traumatic. Do not assume that just because the person is mentally confused or gravely ill, the news is any less upsetting.

Another important matter that will need your immediate attention if the placement comes in an emergency is the appointment of a durable power of attorney or legal guardian for the person. This is a trusted relative, friend, or associate who will speak for the person should he or she be unable to make decisions. Hopefully you, the caregiver, have already been appointed to this position, but if not, do something about it now. Ask the hospital social worker to assist you or call the local Office on Aging for information about this process in your state.

In the crisis placement, you will need to be organized about gathering information. Be prepared to get answers to the following questions when the physician and hospital social worker meet with you and your relative or in a private meeting with you and the social worker:

1. Why is a nursing home necessary? Why can't the person stay in the hospital? Why can't the person be cared for at home? (These are questions you are asking for the patient's benefit.)
2. How much time do you have to find a home?
3. What exactly is the process?
4. What will the hospital staff do to help?

5. What do you need to do and in what order should you do it?
6. What care will be given in the nursing home? Will there be therapy? Will there be special nursing treatments?
7. Is there any possibility this could be a short-term stay; i.e., if the therapy is successful, might the person be able to return to the community?

You may wish to gather this information in a meeting without the patient at first, but do not exclude him or her from the process. It is important to the potential resident's adjustment that he or she be at least a tacit part of the process of finding the home from the outset.

If there is no crisis, you still need to make some personal assessments of the individual situation before you can begin to plan for the possibility of nursing home care. You and your loved one are not exactly like anyone else. While someone else may be at the breaking point, you truly may be capable of managing for some time yet while you seek the nearly perfect home for your relative. While someone else may not be able to deal with the guilt of "putting Mom in a nursing home," you may be able to see the possibilities for an even higher level of caregiving from you once Mom is receiving the daily care she needs professionally.

To understand the level of care needed and, therefore, the most appropriate type of response to those needs, gather the following information:

1. Sit down with the person's physician and any other healthcare professional involved in his or her health care and get an understandable *medical assessment.* What is the diagnosis? What is the prognosis? What treatments are planned and how must they be implemented? (For example, treatments can include medications that you are certainly capable of administering and/or they may include physical or speech or some other type of therapy that must be given by a professional.)
2. On your own or with the help of professionals, make an *assessment of the person's ability to complete basic activities*

of daily living (ADLs) in the situation under which that person now lives. (ADLs include bathing, personal grooming, dressing, toileting, ability to move about without help or with a cane or walker, ability to feed oneself, and ability to shop and prepare meals, if necessary.) What are the needs? How are they being met now? How will they be met if they escalate? *Ask yourself what is needed now that was not needed before?*

3. Next, do a *caregiver's assessment.* In the best situation, the decision to move to a nursing home is up to the older person, but increasingly the decision is made by the primary caregiver and/or family. If more than one family member is involved, there can be conflict, making a decision more complicated. How does each family member feel about the idea of nursing home placement? If some family members are against the idea, what alternatives are they prepared to propose? If there is disagreement among family members, how will the decision be made? Who will speak for the family? This might be an excellent time to consider the services of a case manager.

    Sometimes the decision falls on the primary caregiver—the person who has been providing the bulk of the care needed by the potential nursing home resident. If you are a primary caregiver faced with a decision about nursing home care, you will need to assess your own physical and mental health, your ability to continue to cope, your potential for possibly adding more responsibility and work as this person's primary caregiver, and your chances for success in maintaining this person's lifestyle without irreparable harm to your own. How much time are you giving to caregiving? How much more do you have to give? What facets of your life are being neglected while you give care? In the long run, do you need help to carry on? Could you do a better job of giving loving care to this person if you had some help with the basic care?

4. Take a hard, realistic look at the *financial assessment.* How much does it cost to give care to this person under the present circumstances? Who is paying that bill? At this rate, how long will the money last? Is the person eligible

for public assistance programs that would take the burden of the cost of care off your shoulders as an adult child? If you are a spouse and this person goes to a nursing home, what does that mean for your personal financial situation?

5. Finally, *assess long-term care needs*. As you have seen, sometimes the need is for a relatively short-term care plan—perhaps six months. In other cases, the need is for around-the-clock care that probably will not lessen as time goes on. Using the information you have gathered above, assess the level of care needed.

Do not hesitate to get professional counseling in making these introductory assessments. The chances are good that the climate for making clearheaded decisions on your own is not good right now. Ask questions. Take notes.

What Are the Alternatives?

Nursing home care is expensive. Besides the worry about how expenses will be met, you as the caregiver may go through a guilt period where you wonder whether you had any alternatives to a nursing home. Now is the time for you to find out about those alternatives. The patient, if he or she is capable, may also want to try anything else other than moving into a home.

Once you have a clear assessment of needs, you can consider the options available in the community where the person lives. The chances are good that some or even many of these options have already been tried or are already in place. There is the possibility that adding more services or changing services will solve the problems as well as moving into a nursing home would. So, certainly take some time to consider the possibilities. Begin by completing the following financial data. On the following pages, mark off those services that are already in use, are not possible, or have been tried without success.

MONTHLY

Income:	Expenses:
Salary/wages _____	Rent/mortgage _____
Pension _____	Food _____
IRA/Keogh plan _____	Clothing _____
Annuity _____	Medical _____
Social Security _____	Transportation _____
patient _____	Telephone _____
spouse _____	Utilities _____
Interest on savings _____	Home maintenance _____
Interest on bonds _____	Furnishings _____
Stock dividends _____	Personal items _____
Real estate _____	Insurance _____
Profits from business _____	Taxes _____
Other _____	Other _____
Total income: _____	Total expenses: _____

Housing Needs

What is wrong with where the person lives now? Unsafe? Structurally impossible? (Example: All bedrooms and baths upstairs.) Too isolated? No longer available? (Example: A congregate community that does not permit residents who cannot perform certain tasks independently.)

Now what are the alternatives? Someone living with the person? The person moving in with someone else? A group home (sometimes called board and care or community-based residential facility)? A continuing care or retirement community? A rehabilitation hospital?

Housing needs may be met by:

_____ maintaining the present situation with live-in help (either a hired person or a family member)

_____ moving in with family member

_____ moving into an alternative housing situation (group home, congregate home, rehab hospital, etc.)

Medical/Health Care Needs

What are they and how can they best be met? Is skilled nursing needed in order to perform some special medical treatment? Is therapy needed? Does the person have to be able to go to and from a physician or treatment center? How long will the medical/health care needs be at this level?

Medical/health needs can be met by:

____ in-home nursing and therapy from home care agency

____ outpatient services

____ counseling programs

____ caregiver (hired or family member)

Basic Care Needs

How will the person get meals? Is there a transportation program available to take the person to and from needed medical care appointments? How will the person maintain his or her place of residence? In what phases of personal care (bathing, dressing, toileting, eating) does the person need assistance? How many of these daily care needs are new to the situation if the person has had a sudden or acute health crisis? How many of these needs have in the past been met by the caregiver who is exhausted or too frail to continue to deliver these services?

Basic living needs can be met by:
meals—

____ home-delivered meal program

____ meals taken at a central site (such as a nutrition center or dining room in a congregate situation)

____ caregiver

____ hired help to prepare meals

transportation—

_____ special community program for the older and/or impaired citizen

_____ friends and neighbors

_____ family members

_____ caregiver

home maintenance—

_____ community programs such as homemakers' services, chore services, or handyman programs

_____ hired housekeepers

_____ caregiver

personal care—

_____ home care agency aide

_____ hired help

_____ caregiver

Social Needs

How isolated will the person be? Can he or she participate in programs such as adult daycare? Are there volunteer visiting programs in the community? Can he or she get out to attend religious services, entertainments, and neighborhood functions?

Social and safety needs can be met by:

_____ adult daycare center

_____ outreach programs within the living environment (for example, there are often planned activities in the group or congregate home)

_____ telephone reassurance systems

_____ volunteer visitors

_____ friends and neighbors

_____ family

_____ caregiver

Caregiver Needs

There are at least two lives to be considered here: the patient's and the primary caregiver's. If the caregiver is a spouse, how much of his or her life is enough to sacrifice to the care of this loved one? How much jeopardy is his or her own health in because of excessive caregiving? How many of the other person's needs could be met as well or better by professionals? And if the caregiver is an adult child, how many others are being affected by his or her devotion to an aging parent? Does the caregiver have a spouse? children? How has caregiving affected his or her own physical and mental health?

Caregiver needs may be met by:

_____ finding regular opportunities for taking short and more long-term breaks from caregiving (respite)

_____ engaging the help of other family members to relieve some of the pressures of caregiving

_____ giving up some of the tasks of caregiving to hired services

_____ joining a support group with other caregivers

There is no "grade" on this survey. You are simply gathering information and indicators. For one caregiver, marking a dozen or more of the above indicators may still not mean the nursing home is the best answer. For another caregiver, three or four of the indicators in the right combination may be enough to cause him or her to say, "Yes. It's time to think about it."

Presumably you are left with a short list of options available for continuing to provide care for this older relative within the mainstream of the community. Unless that list answers every need, the chances are that those measures will not be enough and if tried will simply be a stopgap means of stalling for time until a more permanent solution can be found.

It is when you have tried everything and every combination of things and that still is not enough that the decision to look for a nursing home may come fully into play. And that is difficult. You are proud that you have coped for so long. You have always been able to manage until now, and it is tough to give up without giving it one more try. But into some households comes that moment of truth when the only answer—indeed the most loving answer—is the nursing home. And this moment is going to be unique to each family. One person in the family may advocate for "Now." Someone else may insist the decision can wait. The older person may be saying something else altogether.

How Do You Talk to Your Relative?

Americans caring for their older relatives are faced with a dilemma. On the one hand, one out of every five older persons will need the kind of care provided in a nursing home at some time in their lives. On the other hand, there is the "fear factor"—the belief based on half-recalled reports about abuse or poor care that any nursing home experience is going to be terrible. Where do you begin?

Breaking the News

The chances are good that your relative, regardless of the level of mental competency, has some pretty well ingrained attitudes about life in a nursing home. The chances are also good that the person is not particularly receptive to the idea. One caregiver told the story of her mother, a person in the later stages of Alzheimer's disease, who when she walked into the nursing home and realized that her daughter had brought her there to live literally tried to escape. She raced up and down the corridor, banged on doors and windows, and shouted to anyone she saw that she was being kidnapped and held against her will.

Many caregivers recall conversations in better days with their relatives about nursing homes. Some of them promised "never"—never to put the person in one of "those places." Some of them recall being met with silence that said as eloquently as any words, "I do not wish to discuss this possibility—ever." And now the physician or some other professional is urging them (perhaps even writing orders for them) to take this hard step.

The ideal situation is one in which both the patient and the caregiver have discussed the possibility of a need for nursing home care at some point; in which the patient and the caregiver have visited others who live in nursing homes and know the general routine and style of living; and in which both parties have spent some time making plans, thinking about choices, and gathering information that will be needed.

The ideal situation, however, is almost never the real situation.

In the event of an emergency placement, let the professional broach the subject. If the older person is in the hospital, let the physician, discharge planner, and/or social worker do the hard work. You should be there when this conversation takes place, but the words need not come from your mouth. If there is going to be anger and recrimination, let it be toward these others who will not be a part of the ongoing picture.

Why be there at all, then? Because you need to hear the same words the older person hears. It is too easy for those words to get twisted in translation: "Did the doctor talk to you today, Mom?" "Yes." "About a nursing home?" "Oh that. He said one of these days . . . ." You know he didn't say "one of these days," he said "today," but how do you call her on it if you weren't there?

Another reason for being there is so that you can phrase questions that may be on the person's mind but may remain unasked. Some physicians are notoriously poor communicators and older patients are notoriously reluctant to "bother the doctor." So you need to put the questions into words. "Why can't the care be given at home?" "Can we hire someone to do that at home?" And if there is a chance that this could be a short-term stay, clarify that possibility. "If the therapy is successful and Mom makes the kind of progress you are suggesting, could she come home?" Certainly the doctor will not make promises, but if indeed this is a potential short-term stay you want the patient to understand that fact and use it as incentive.

Working through the Initial Shock

Once the news has been given, your work begins in earnest. Possibly the reaction you will get is no reaction. Your relative will close off from the discussion, refusing to express any emotion at all. Many caregivers are surprised at this attitude of apathy when they were expecting anger and gnashing of teeth. But silence can mean the emotions are just as deeply felt as they would be if they were expressed aloud. It may also mean that the person does not know what to say or ask.

Your role becomes one of trying to elicit some of those feelings or at least of trying to express some sympathy and understanding. Think about what might be going through the mind of an individual who has just been informed that he or she needs to take up residence in a nursing home:

- "Don't call it 'home'—it's an institution."
- "I have to move to a much smaller place—probably share a room; what will happen to all my beautiful and special things?"
- "I'll be in there with all those sick old people."
- "My family will go on without me and will be too busy to come and see me."
- "I'll be locked up there. Oh, I never thought this would happen to me."
- "I've managed my own affairs all my life, now this. I don't want some twenty-year-old telling me when to get up and where I can go."
- "People don't get better in nursing homes."
- "My life is ending."
- "I'll die there."

Expressed or not, the person is going to go through several stages of adjustment to the idea. At this point, he or she is having to come to terms with the need for nursing home care. Once the need has been recognized (though not always accepted), the person moves on to stage two: coping with the ramifications of residency in a nursing home: loss of status in the community, loss of territory in the form of a home and furnishings and possessions, loss of contact with neighbors and friends and even family, loss of autonomy and freedom to make choices about some of the most basic aspects of life. Once the person actually moves into the home, there are still further stages of adjustment to make.

On the other hand, while emotions may run deep for both you and the patient, try not to anticipate. One caregiver who thought her mother was devastated at the news found out her mother's greatest concern was that a home would be chosen for her on the other side of town from the place she had lived for years. Once she was assured that homes were available in her old neighborhood, she settled into the adjustment process rather quickly.

Take your cues from the patient. If things seem to be going well, offer ample opportunity for expression of feelings and concerns but do not go digging. And do not project your own concerns and guilts onto the patient. One caregiver was so consumed with the idea that her mother might be abused in the home that she went overboard in trying to convince her mother that there was little chance such a thing would happen. In her zeal, she created an issue her mother had given little thought to and became terrified of.

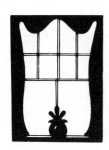

Chapter 3

Paying for Care in a Nursing Home

You need to know that care in a nursing home is costly. According to *Consumer Reports* (May 1988, p. 300), "A year in a nursing home now costs on average $22,000 or more. By the year 2018, it will cost about $55,000 if inflation stays at recent moderate rates."

Nursing home care includes in a quoted daily rate some standard services such as room, meals, linens, and custodial and nursing care, and it often involves extras such as therapy, care by a physician, and medications, which must be paid for in addition to the daily rate. As of this writing, what is covered as "basic" varies from state to state and usually home to home. It is vital that you understand from the outset what will be included in the daily rate and what will not.

Every potential nursing home resident and his or her caregiver needs to be concerned about costs. Even if the bill is to be covered in part or in whole by federal assistance programs such as Medicare and Medicaid, you need to make certain that you clearly understand the rules when it comes to who pays for what. The cost of care in a nursing home is based on how much care is required and how many services are used.

The other factor that can influence cost and thus the choice of one home over another is the length of stay factor. If the person's doctor indicates that the stay could be for a relatively short period of time and will primarily be for rehabilitative purposes, Medicare may cover a part of the

costs. In that case, you will definitely want to choose a home
that is Medicare-certified.

You need to understand that payment source is a major
factor in choosing a home or having a home available to you.
While a nursing home cannot discriminate against a Title
XIX (Medicaid) resident once he or she moves into the home,
the facility can refuse to accept the person in the first place
unless specific state statutes prohibit such refusal.

Remember, as the primary caregiver, you would be wise
to seek some immediate advice (if you have not already done
so) on the process of appointing a durable power of attorney
for your relative. You also need to collect all insurance,
Medicare, Title XIX (Medicaid) (if applicable), and Social
Security identification and carry them with you. The home
you choose will need to photocopy these documents.

If you are a spouse considering the possibility of a nursing
home for your husband or wife, you need to understand that
your *joint* assets must be available to pay for nursing home
care until those assets have been spent down to a minimal
level. Recent legislation has raised those minimums
somewhat, but impoverishment of the spouse who remains
in the community is still a very real problem in long-term
care (see page 34).

Aside from costs, you and your relative may need to be
concerned about availability of space. A 1988 federal report
on issues of long-term care notes that each state varies in
the number of available beds for every 1,000 members of the
over-75 age population. A nationwide check of Medicaid-
certified nursing home beds in 1985 found that numbers of
total beds ranged all the way from about 200 beds per 1000
in Minnesota to around 60 beds per 1000 in Florida. On top
of that, the report found a 91 percent occupancy rate of those
available beds to be the national average. One reason for this
"tight supply" indicator is that many states have taken steps
to limit the number of available beds for Medicaid patients
in an effort to control expenses. As a result, some nursing
homes may admit patients who have the ability to pay
privately or whose care needs are relatively simple ahead of
those who need heavy skilled care and/or public support for

care. Those who may have to wait longest for admittance to a nursing home according to the report are those "(1) with mental/behavioral problems, (2) with multiple . . . dependencies requiring extra nursing care, and (3) financed by Medicaid."[1]

In the long run, everything comes down to costs—for both federal and state governments as well as for the potential resident and his or her family. In 1985, the bill for long-term care nationally was $45 billion. (Long-term care includes both nursing home care and home or community care.) The Congressional Budget Office predicts that expenditures for long-term care could increase by as much as 200 percent in the next 10 years, based on current costs plus increased numbers of older persons plus increased service needs of that population.

Of the $45 billion spent in 1985, a whopping $36 billion (or 80 percent of the total expenditure) went to pay for nursing home care. Next to expenditures for hospitals and physicians, nursing home care is the third largest health expenditure in the national budget.

Examine Payment Sources

There are four common sources of payment for 90+ percent of nursing home care. The rest is paid for from miscellaneous sources. You will do yourself a favor if you take a moment now to understand each in more detail.

Medicare
It is astonishing how many otherwise well-educated and knowledgeable people (including some physicians) still believe that Medicare will foot the bill for nursing home care. In order to set the record straight, here are the conditions under which Medicare will contribute any funds to care in a nursing home:

---

[1]"Long Term Care for the Elderly: Issues of Need, Access and Cost," report to Chairman, Subcommittee on Health and Long Term Care, Select Committee on Aging, House of Representatives, November 1988, p. 22.

Medicare pays for up to 150 days of skilled nursing home care following at least a three-day hospitalization where the patient needs skilled nursing and/or rehabilitative care under a doctor's orders with the clear possibility of improvement. From day 1–8, Medicare will pay all but $25.50 per day. For days 9–150, Medicare pays everything if services are required. You need to understand that just because Medicare pays *up to* 150 days does not necessarily mean your relative is eligible for the full 150 days. After day 150, Medicare pays nothing.

According to the U.S. Department of Health and Human Services, ". . . Medicare will not pay for care in a skilled nursing home *unless the patient needs skilled nursing care or skilled rehabilitation services on a daily basis. Medicare cannot pay for care . . . if the care needed is mainly custodial.*" Residents may "demand billing" if they are denied Medicare status upon entering the nursing home. This means that the resident has the right to request the home to submit the bill to Medicare and let Medicare determine whether or not the bill is covered. If you are a caregiving spouse, this may be especially important to you because if Medicare does pay part of the bill, you are preserving private funds for a while longer. You should also know that *each* hospitalization may qualify the resident for Medicare aid.

All caregivers need to keep in mind, however, that as of this writing, Medicare pays less that 2 percent of all nursing home costs.

Private Insurance

A number of insurance companies are showing an overdue interest in offering policies for long-term care. Such policies are expensive, are based on age and prior conditions of illness, either chronic or acute, and are not generally owned by today's older population. Most policies have clauses that prohibit coverage for any condition that existed prior to enrollment in the plan and many exclude from coverage Alzheimer's or other illnesses that result in mental impairment.

Unless your relative has such a policy, the chances are that it is already too late for such a policy to do much good in terms of helping your relative pay for nursing home care. If, however, you are planning ahead you may want to investigate the idea of purchasing long-term care insurance. If so, use the following guidelines:

- Evaluate and compare several programs and policies.
- Look for restrictions that limit benefits such as long waiting periods, limitations on benefit periods, and exclusion of specific illnesses (such as Alzheimer's disease).
- Make certain the policy covers all levels of long-term care including home care, skilled nursing care, and custodial care.
- Inquire whether the policy is guaranteed renewable for life and whether or not the premium will vary with age and disability.
- Seek the opinion of such objective agencies as the office of the State Insurance Commissioner, the local Office on Aging, or the ombudsperson.

Insurance for long-term care is a new area of funding and is changing almost daily. Consumers are advised to keep their eyes and ears open and collect information as it becomes available. Coverage as well as premium rates could improve dramatically in a very short time. As of this writing, private insurance covers only about 1 percent of nursing home costs.

Personal Funds

The greatest amount of the bill for nursing home care is covered by the personal funds of the residents. The care is expensive, and it does not take long to "spend down" those sums, but the fact is that older people in need of care pay for that care to the tune of 51.4 percent per year.

As the caregiver, you will want to take a good look at your relative's finances as far in advance of the possible need for nursing home care as is feasible. Funds that are unavailable without the payment of fines or loss of interest such as those in certificates of deposit are still fair game for paying the nursing home. Stocks, real estate (other than the personal home if the spouse is still living there), bonds—all are expected to be liquidated as the need arises.

By planning ahead, you may be able to protect some assets. This is mainly done for the protection of the spouse who still is healthy and will remain in the family home and neighborhood. Without protection of assets, this person can become impoverished although some progress is being made to correct this scandal. As of September 30, 1989, spouses of persons who reside in a nursing home and whose care is paid for by Medicaid will be permitted to keep one-half of all the couple's assets, or $12,000, whichever is greater (up to a maximum of $60,000). The spouse who remains at home can also retain a monthly income of at least 122 percent of the federal poverty level for couples ($786 a month in 1989).

If you are giving care to a spouse who may become a nursing home resident, call your state Office on Aging and ask if there are any special provisions to prevent spousal impoverishment.

Medicaid, or Title XIX

This is a federally funded but state-managed program to provide health care for persons of all ages who cannot afford care themselves. The older person in the nursing home typically uses up his or her assets and then applies for assistance from Medicaid. The Title XIX or Medicaid program currently pays for 41.8 percent of the care given older persons in nursing homes.

Since standards for Medicaid eligibility are established by individual states, contact your local Office on Aging, state Office on Aging, Social Security office, or ombudsperson program (see Appendix A, pages 156-160) to determine eligibility require-ments within your relative's state.

You and the nursing home admissions counselor should be very clear about what the payment sources will be, how it might change, and when it might change. You will want clear, written information about any policies that can affect your relative if he or she goes from private payment to Medicaid. Any clarifications you can get in writing will serve you later on if there is a problem. Also check with the ombudsperson in the area and get him or her to give you a written statement of policy regarding these matters so you know what can and cannot be done in terms of Medicaid. In spite of the laws on the books, Medicaid discrimination is a national problem. Do not be naive about this. Find out the facts about your state's rules concerning rights of Title XIX (Medicaid) residents.

REMEMBER:

1. Understand the Basics

Costs will vary from one home to another; at this writing, basic services are not standardized.

Billing procedures also differ, making it sometimes difficult to really compare costs between homes.

Nearly every home has a basic monthly charge and then adds charges for what that home considers to be additional services.

Usually, the basic charge covers room, meals, housekeeping, linen (not personal laundry), general nursing care and activities, personal or custodial care, and medical record-keeping.

"Extras" (services for which there is an additional charge) often include services by physicians beyond those required by law, including ophthalmologists, dentists, and podiatrists; medications; rehabilitative therapy; laboratory work; X rays and other diagnostic services; and personal care services such as personal laundry and beautician and barber services. (Sometimes a special diet may be considered an "extra," as may having help with feeding or bathing.)

According to the nursing home reforms enacted in 1987, the nursing home cannot require you as a family member to sign a contract agreeing to guarantee or pay as a third party for care for a defined period of time before the resident starts to receive Title XIX (Medicaid).

Your relative's and/or your ability to meet costs out of pocket may play a role in whether or not the home is willing to accept this person as a resident. (Even a home certified for Medicaid can refuse to accept a person who is coming into the home under the Title XIX pay source.)

If you are a caregiving spouse, you must spend your joint assets to cover costs of care before that person becomes eligible for public assistance such as Medicaid. (See page 33.)

2. Collect Financial Data

Gather the person's Social Security card, Medicare card, Title XIX (Medicaid) card, if applicable, and all other insurance as well as veterans' and pension benefits information in one place. This information will be needed when you decide on a nursing home.

Fill out the following financial statement to ascertain what assets are available and what your relative's financial situation is.

Name: _____

Social Security number: _____

Medicare number: _____

Supplemental insurance number: _____

Title XIX (Medicaid) number (if applicable): _____

Income sources:
   Social Security $ _____ per _____

   Pension $ _____ per _____

   Annuity $ _____ per _____

   Interest $ _____ per _____

   Dividends $ _____ per _____

   Income from other sources $ _____ per _____

Total annual income $ _____

Assets:
   Real estate
   (estimated market value) $ _____

   Checking accounts
   Bank: $ _____

Bank: $ _____

Savings accounts
Bank: $ _____

Bank: $ _____

Other investments (certificates of deposit, IRA accounts, etc.)

Where located: Amount:

_____

_____

_____

Life insurance

Company: Value:

_____

_____

_____

Liabilities: (List any financial obligations owed by the person with amounts):

_____

_____

_____

Once you have collected this information, the hospital discharge planner, nursing home admissions counselor, or county or state social worker can help you determine what the pay source will be.

If assets are substantial and nursing home care is not an immediate need but may be a consideration for the future, get some financial and legal advice from your attorney or financial planner, especially if you are a caregiving spouse.

Unless you already know, you will need to call and find out if a facility is certified to accept Medicare and/or Medicaid payments before you tour the home if either of those will figure into your funding plans.

When you tour, be sure you get a clear statement in writing of what is and is not covered in the basic care fee. Also get a written and itemized list of charges for items not covered under basic care.

When you are in the final selection process, do not let items that will not be a factor in your relative's care play a role in your decision. For example, if the home's basic rate includes physical therapy and your relative does not need such therapy, that is not a plus. On the other hand, if the home offers mental health counseling for a separate fee and your relative has some chronic depression, that factor could very well be important to the selection process.

3. Understand Costs

Nursing homes have two categories of charges:

- daily rates for room, board, and some nursing services
- extra charges for *anything* that is not specifically covered in the daily rate (personal laundry, therapies, use of wheelchair or other supportive device, ancillary medical services such as dental care, etc.).

Nursing homes certified for either Medicaid or Medicare are required to furnish the resident with complete information about both the daily rate and any extra charges. You will probably receive this information when you tour the home. If you do not, ask for it before you leave. You must have this information if you are using any form of supplemental pay source (private insurance, Medicare, or Medicaid) in order to find out what the supplemental pay source will and will not cover.

As of this writing, some costs may be influenced by the level of care under which a resident is admitted to the home. Until at least 1990, facilities will be designated as "skilled nursing facilities" (SNF), and "intermediate care facilities" (ICF). Some nursing homes may be certified for both levels of care.

The differences have to do with the level of nursing care required. For example, in the area of feeding, a resident who simply needs help eating with a spoon or fork would be intermediate level care while someone who required tube feedings would be skilled level care. Likewise, someone who required only routine skin care in the form of regular assessment and basic care would be intermediate level, while someone who required regularly prescribed treatments for a skin disorder would be skilled level. Generally speaking, if the person's condition is medically complicated and unstable, that resident would need a skilled nursing facility. Someone whose care needs were more basic and stable would be termed an intermediate care resident.

Having read all that, you need to know that if the nursing home reforms enacted in 1987 proceed on schedule there will be no differentiation after 1990—all homes will be certified on the basis of offering skilled care.

When your relative moves into the home, he or she (or you as legal guardian) will be asked to sign a number of documents. One of the most important of these is the admissions agreement or contract. This legally binding pact is discussed more fully on pages 84-85. For now, you need only be aware of its existence and make a note to yourself to be certain that what you have been told is what actually is written in this contract.

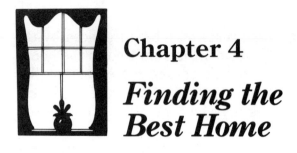

Chapter 4

Finding the Best Home

The news has been given to your older relative. You and that person have each dealt in at least some preliminary manner with the myriad of emotions and reactions that accompany the idea of nursing homes. You have gathered the financial information necessary to select a home. It is time to find the right home. Now the real work begins.

In the emergency placement, the hospital discharge planner or case manager will give you a list of some homes that are available to meet the care and financial needs of your relative. Visit every home suggested to you by the professionals—usually three to four homes. (If you are doing the placement basically on your own under emergency circumstances, prescreen all the homes people suggest to you and then tour the three to four that seem most suitable.)

If a home you have considered is not on the list, ask why. Possibly that home is not certified to accept Medicare or Medicaid (if either of those pay sources apply), there is no bed available, or the home does not offer the level of nursing care your relative needs. For these reasons, you will just be spinning your wheels and wasting valuable time if you go off on your own and try to find a suitable home. Remember: The social services staff is there to help you—let them. On the other hand, if the staff can give no valid reason for not considering the home, check it out anyway. Social services professionals are human and bound to have their own biases about which homes might be appropriate.

Of the homes suggested, you may need to consider the best choice between the small home and the larger one. (Nursing home size is rated in number of beds: 100 beds or less is a small home; from 100 to 150 is a medium-sized facility; large homes can have 300 or more beds.) If your relative's stay could be short-term for therapy and rehabilitation, those departments are more important to consider than other facets of the home may be. If your relative is going to live there permanently and is fairly active, programming and residential amenities are more important. And if your relative is gravely ill, nursing care is primary.

What a Nursing Home Does

Before you can take an intelligent look at any facility, you need to know what it is supposed to offer. Basically, a nursing home offers a resident care. Services fall into three broad categories: medical care, residential (sometimes called custodial) care, and social care. Regardless of location or size, there are a number of common services a resident may expect.

Medical Care

Common medical care services include the following:

1. A physician is on call for the home (or the person can choose his or her own personal physician) and sees residents on a regular basis. The doctor is not in all the time. He or she makes rounds at the home. One of the standard misconceptions about life in a nursing home is that the doctor will always be available or at least to the extent he or she is in a hospital. Remember, a nursing home is not a hospital.
2. In a nursing home, *nursing* is the key word. Residents are served by nursing staff at three levels: the registered nurse (RN) who provides supervision and administration for all nursing services within the home and provides the highly skilled care that is sometimes called for, the licensed practical nurse (LPN, or LVN in some states) who handles the less skilled nursing tasks usually providing a good deal

of the bedside care, and the nursing assistant (aide) who by some estimates provides as much as 90 percent of the actual hands-on care given in nursing homes.

3. Depending on their size, location, and certification, nursing homes may either have in-house rehabilitative and therapy services or contract for such services to come in from an outside agency. These services include physical therapy, occupational therapy, and speech therapy. (Recreational therapy is a part of the medical plan but will be covered below under social care.) Frequently, such services, with the exception of recreational therapy, are not included in the daily rate.

4. In light of DRGs (see page 4) and the restrictions they set for length of hospital stays, many nursing homes today are providing the kind of acute care once given only in hospitals.

5. Services such as dental care, podiatry care, optometrist services, pharmaceutical services, and laboratory services are available but usually not covered in the daily rate. Supplies and equipment such as diapers, special nutritional supplements, special mattresses, and possibly ambulatory devices such as wheelchairs also may not be covered.

Residential Care

Common residential care services include the following:

1. Each home by law offers a safety and security plan that includes an evacuation plan in the event of emergency as well as safety features within the home such as heavy fire doors, an emergency sprinkler system, call bells for alerting staff in the event of emergency, handrails along hallways, and lighting and other design features that maximize safety.

2. Residents are to be provided with meals that are nutritious and palatable, planned and prepared by a trained staff with attention given to special diets (diabetic, for example) and special needs (such as food that must be pureed for those who cannot chew well).

3. Each resident is entitled to have his or her own space within the home—usually a room shared with one other person

although some homes offer private rooms or rooms shared by three persons. In that space, state and federal regulations mandate certain standard furnishings be provided: usually a bed, closet, dresser, bedside table, and chair. These furnishings do not leave much room for personal belongings or keepsakes.

4. The home provides laundry services, linens, and house-keeping and maintenance services to every resident. These services are not reimburseable under Medicaid or public assistance programs in most states so the home can decide to what extent services will be provided.
5. Residents are entitled to assistance with personal care if necessary. Staff can assist the person to eat, bathe, get to and from the bathroom, dress, and transfer from one position to another.

Social Care
Common social care services include the following:

1. Since the nursing home resident is just that—a resident of this rather closed community—the home provides a program of recreational and social opportunities.
2. Staffing at a home may include persons trained to conduct recreational activities such as crafts, games, parties, outings, and entertainments. It may also include the services of a trained social worker who can assist the resident with any problems he or she may be having within the home or with his or her family.
3. Many homes have a small in-house commercial community that may include a barber/beauty shop, a soda shop, a gift shop, postal services, and/or a restaurant. Such services are not included in the daily rate.
4. Every home must offer the opportunity for the residents to organize a resident council with elected representatives who can speak out for the residents. In recent years, the addition of a family council made up of caregivers and family members has been added in many homes.
5. Every home also offers the presence of other people—staff and other residents. For a person who has become somewhat isolated in his or her own home, losing contact

with friends and neighbors, rarely getting out, this can mean the opportunity for social contact, an important factor of health at any age.

If you are planning for the possibility of nursing home care and there is no emergency, call or write the state department of health and request a listing of nursing homes in the area where the person lives. Talk to friends, neighbors, other family members, and any other people you know who have had some experience with particular homes for their recommendations. Call the office of the ombudsperson. Check the yellow pages of your telephone directory. Do not try to consider every home (unless you live in an area where there are only a few choices). Make a list of four to six homes and begin.

Take location into consideration in making your list. Remember, it may be more important for the nursing home to be located in an area convenient for the family to visit than in the resident's old neighborhood.

What to Find Out before You Tour

Using the information gathered in your assessment of your relative, make a list of needs. (What you are listing here is every requirement that *must* be met by the home you choose. You cannot compromise on these issues.)

Medical/Nursing/Therapy Needs
(Example: 1. Person needs physical therapy every day. 2. Person needs a special dressing or treatment performed by a nurse. 3. Person needs complete skilled nursing care.)

1.
2.
3.

Financial Needs
(Example: 1. Home must be certified for Title XIX (Medicaid). 2. Home must be certified for Medicare. 3. Home must offer as complete a package as possible under basic care.)

1.
2.
3.

Social/Custodial Needs

(Example: 1. Person needs help feeding self. 2. Person needs help with dressing and grooming. 3. Person wanders and needs watching.)

1.
2.
3.

Prescreening by Telephone

Some facilities can be eliminated by information you can gather without visiting the home. Using the questions below, screen each home on your list by telephone.

1. Is the home licensed or certified by the state, meaning the state regularly inspects the home? If the home is not licensed or certified, it is not eligible to receive Medicare and/or Medicaid funding and is not inspected on a regular basis. Is the administrator licensed? (If the answer is no to either of these questions, consider crossing this home off the list and not even pursuing the rest of the questions.)
2. What level of care is provided? (Until 1989, homes might be described as "skilled nursing facilities" or "intermediate care facilities." After 1989, all will be skilled care.)
3. Do they accept Medicare? Medicaid? VA benefits? (The pay source may be a more deciding factor in your selection process than you might think. If the person's care can be partially met by Medicare, you need a home certified for that purpose. If your relative will eventually need Medicaid funds, you also need to choose a home certified to receive those funds.)
4. What happens when personal funds are exhausted and public pay sources are needed?
5. How many residents can the home accommodate? Is there a vacancy available?

6. If not, is there a waiting list? How long is the waiting list?
7. What are the rates? What is included? What is extra?
8. Is an advance deposit required? How much?
9. What are the billing procedures and payment policies?
10. Are there other admittance requirements?
11. Are the special services needed available (therapy, special diet, etc.)?
12. What hospital does the home's physician send residents to in the event of a need for hospitalization?
13. If you plan to use the facility's staff physician, who is this person and what is his or her reputation? Talk to family members of residents currently in the home.
14. What is the ratio of nursing staff (including aides who provide the vast majority of care) to residents? A ratio of 1 to 5 for the day shift, 1 to 7 for evenings, and 1 to 10 for nights has been recommended as a guideline.[1]
15. Does the home have a social worker on staff? The nursing home reforms of 1987 mandate that every facility serving 120 residents or more must have at least one full-time social worker. What is the ratio of social workers to residents. (This will give you some idea of where the home places its priorities.)
16. How many years has senior staff been there? Ask the administrator or admissions counselor.
17. Who owns the home? How long has it been owned by these persons? Are they a local group? If not, where are their headquarters? How many homes do they own?
18. What is the history of the home? How has it grown?
19. What is the level of training for the administrative staff? for the director of nursing? for the director of social services?
20. Does the home have any recent history of serious code violations or complaints? (This is an issue you will

---

[1]C. Bennett, *What It Is and What It Could Be* (New York: The Tiresias Press, 1980).

eventually address to the ombudsperson, but it does not hurt to bring the matter up just to see the response you get.)

Use the following chart to summarize what you learn after each call.

Nursing Home

	A	B	C	D	E
Home has current license	✓				
Home is certified for Medicare	✓				
Home is certified for Medicaid	✓				
Administrator is licensed	✓				
Home has bed available					
Home has waiting list	✓				
Home can meet all special care needs of patient (diet, therapy, skilled nursing procedures)	✓				
Home has no recent history of serious code violations/ complaints	✓				
Home is convenient for resident's physician	✓				
Home is convenient for visits by family					
Home's location is appealing to patient	✓				

	A	B	C	D	E
Home has _?_ residents	130				
Home is connected to relative's religion	✓				
Home is nonprofit	✓				
Home is privately owned					
Home is locally owned	✓				
Home is owned by national corporation					

When this chart is completed, you may have already crossed off one or more homes. Your next step is to call the ombudsperson in your area (see list in Appendix A, pages 156–160) and find out if there are any outstanding problems with any of the homes you have left on the list. In this case, the ombudsperson program serves as a kind of Better Business Bureau in that they can only tell you if they have received complaints and how those complaints have been addressed in the past. Many states have a toll-free number for the ombudsperson program.

The state of Illinois instituted a ratings program similar to a travel club's "star" system. They rate their homes with stars: no stars for the worst, six stars for the best. They call the program QUIP (Quality Incentive Program), and they back up their ratings program with rigorous standards and spot inspections and a cash bonus for star-winners—twenty-five cents per patient per day for each star earned. The plan is a winner on several fronts not the least of which is its emphasis on the positive nature of the nursing home rather than the negative.

Via a computer network available through the state department of health services, California residents can screen nursing homes for deficiencies, complaints, and citations received over the previous two years. Similar programs that make information more readily available to consumers are being introduced in other states. Call your state Office on Aging for special information services that may be available.

Finally, your prescreening process should include talking to anyone who might have some additional knowledge of the homes left on your list—neighbors, friends, other family members, etc.

This sounds like a lot of work but should just mean an hour or so on the phone. The person you wish to speak to at the home is the admissions director. If the home meets your basic needs, go ahead and schedule an appointment to tour the home while you have the person on the phone. If for some reason you decide not to tour, you can always cancel.

What to Look for on Tour

Chapter 5 includes a complete checklist for you to use as you tour each home. The checklist covers all the facets of nursing home residency. Some of the information asked for in this checklist will not be applicable to your relative, but much of it will be. Before you turn to the checklist, read the following material so that you are prepared to make the most of your tour.

When you tour the home, pay attention to four key areas: the physical plant, the services, the residents, and the staff.

General Observations

Your tour begins the minute you walk up to the door. What does the outside of the building tell you about the place? How do the grounds look? How well maintained is the exterior of the building? How safe and convenient are the entrances and exits to and from the building?

Open the door and walk in. Stop. What is your first impression of what you see before you? Listen. What do you hear? What should you hear? Sniff. What do you smell?

Do not be sold on flashy packaging. Many homes have gorgeous lobbies and grounds that could qualify for a design award. But your relative is not coming just to sit in the lobby or out on the patio. Your relative is possibly going to live here, with these other residents and with the staff who provide their care.

How are you received by the first person from the staff with whom you have contact? (This may be a receptionist.) How are you received by the person who is to lead your tour? Have your requests for meeting key personnel been honored? Who seems to be setting the pace for the tour—you or the guide?

Physical Plant

The tour will most likely start in the lobby. Nursing homes commonly put a lot of effort and money into making this area attractive. But again do not be taken in by good decorating. If the area is clearly intended to be used as a gathering place, are there residents confined by the space? Is it convenient and safe for wheelchairs and walkers? Tile floors may be less inviting than thick carpeting, but they are much easier to move a wheelchair or walker across. On the other hand, tile floors can be a problem if a resident has a fall. Happily some carpeting designs that serve both the mobility and safety needs of residents are available. Are the furnishings geared to the residents in terms of comfort and safety? Many nursing homes design their lobby area not for the older person who will live there, but for the families who are the most likely to be impressed by such trappings. What about a secure area outdoors where residents can sit in warmer weather and gather for special events?

If your guide shows you one resident room on one floor and comments that "the other wings are just like this one," ask if your relative will be on that wing, in that room. If not, ask to see other resident rooms in other wings on other floors. In the case of the emergency placement, assuming the home has said it has a room available, you should be able to see not only the actual room but meet the roommate as well, if there is one.

Note the arrangement of the room and its furnishings. Is there a window? Are furnishings geared to the residents?

(Example: Are mirrors hung to be usable by someone who is seated?) Is there adequate closet space, drawer space, and lighting? Where is the bathroom? Are there call bells (to summon emergency help) by the bed and in the bathroom? In shared rooms, what efforts are made to ensure each resident some personal privacy? Are there signs of personal touches in the rooms you visit? If not, ask how long the person has lived in that room. In short, observe what attempts have been made to give the resident control over his or her environment.

In the public areas of the home (lounges, dining rooms, hallways), are details geared to the resident who is frail and impaired? Look for wide doorways that easily accommodate wheelchairs and walkers, elevator buttons and light switches that are accessible to persons in wheelchairs or with physical impairments, and signage that makes it easy for persons with visual problems and confusion to find their way. Look for signs that tell you the home's administration has made an effort to assist residents to live as independently and with as much dignity as possible.

While you are looking at the rooms, ask how the nursing home decides who will be rooming with whom. Ask how many of the beds in the home are currently occupied. (Most good homes run at capacity or near capacity all the time.) If the rooms shown to you are either private or semiprivate rooms, ask if there are any cases where more than two persons share a room. How many people share a bathroom? Are call lights within easy reach of persons in bed? As you walk through the home, note whether or not call lights are answered within a reasonable time.

Medical Services

You are considering the idea of a nursing home because your relative needs more care or other available options than you can provide at the moment. You need to keep in mind that your chief concern is your relative's care and lifestyle. You may be impressed with the programs that take residents out into the community for concerts and other events, but if your relative will be mostly in bed and unable to leave the home, opportunities for field trips should not enter into your screening process.

Every resident of a nursing home must be under the care of a physician. The new nursing home reform act (see Appendix B, page 161) requires that every resident in a nursing home be allowed to select his or her own personal physician. You and/or your relative may decide that being under the care of the home's staff physician is the best idea. If so, make certain that you meet this physician either when you tour the home (make it known in advance that you wish to meet the physician) or at a separate time in his or her office. Ask questions about the physician's routine. How often does the physician visit each resident? Does he or she actually see the resident and review records each time? How long has this doctor been on the staff? Is he or she the physician for other homes?

You need other information about medical care as well. What are the home's procedures in the event of a medical emergency? What are the arrangements for making emergency transfer to a hospital? Which hospital?

Tour the nurses' station. This is headquarters for the nursing staff in a particular wing. Ask how many residents are cared for from that station. Ask to see the room where medications are stored and prepared for distribution. Look for orderliness and security. If your relative will need any special nursing care, ask detailed questions about how and by whom that care will be given.

Ask questions about the level of nursing staffing. Who is in charge on each shift? an RN? LPN? How often is training updated through inservices? Are there any incentive programs for staff members (in all departments) for outstanding job performance and caregiving?

The nursing home reforms of 1987 mandate that a licensed nurse be on duty at all times and that a registered nurse be on duty for at least one eight-hour shift every day of the year including weekends and holidays. *But the quality of care your relative will receive cannot be measured simply in number of staff available. It is far more critical that you pay attention as you tour to details such as staff-resident interaction, resident appearance, and staff attitudes.*

Pay special attention to the nursing assistants or aides. These are the people who will provide most of the care your relative will need. Ask your tour guide about their training, their opportunities for advancement, their longevity on the job, and incentives for better performance. If the tour guide cannot answer such questions, direct them to the adminis- trator. Sometimes there is a need for an older person to be restrained either chemically (by medication) or physically (by use of a restrictive soft belt). The nursing home reform act states that such restraint may not take place without a clear *medical* reason for the restraint and certainly never for the simple convenience of the staff in handling the resident.

While restraints of any type seem like harsh measures and certainly add to the negative image of the nursing home, restraints are sometimes very necessary. One example would be the case where a person has lost motor control and is in danger of falling from his or her chair even while sitting passively. In this case, a doctor may prescribe a soft cloth belt tied around the waist and the chair to hold the resident in the chair. Another example is the Alzheimer's resident who in his or her confusion constantly attempts to leave the home. In such a case, the physician may prescribe medication to calm the anxieties of the confused person.

However, any restraint must be prescribed by a doctor and must be used *only* to protect the health and/or safety of the resident. Look around as you tour and observe residents who have been physically restrained. How are they doing? How frequently are they being checked by staff members? Does the restraint seem excessively tight or binding? Does the person seem to accept the restraint? Do you see signs of overmedication and excessive sedation? Can you see the reason for the restraint? If not, perhaps you could ask and see what sort of explanation you get. The answer could give you some insight into the attitudes and the philosophy of the home's staff.

Rehabilitative Services

Medical care in a nursing home encompasses a range of endeavors beyond the realm of doctors and nurses. In the case of almost every resident, medical care includes one or more of the following therapies:

- physical therapy—exercises and treatments to rehabilitate a person's ability to move more independently
- occupational therapy—exercises and counseling to assist the person in regaining basic skills in activities of daily living such as self-feeding, shaving, grooming, etc.; may also include arts and crafts that assist the person in achieving a sense of accomplishment—see recreational therapy below
- speech therapy—exercises and treatments to assist the person in regaining speech patterns when possible and in communicating with reduced speech when rehab is not possible
- recreational therapy—activities that help the person to achieve a higher quality of life satisfaction within the necessary confines of an institutional environment; activities may include educational programs, cards, songfests, crafts, clubs, outings, parties, etc. (Remember: You are not choosing activities for yourself; you are looking at them from the viewpoint of your relative.)

Ask to visit each therapy department if it is in session. Ask if rehabilitative therapies such as physical and speech therapy are provided in-house (the therapists are on staff) or by an outside agency. Ask for a copy of the month's recreational activity schedule. Note the types of activities listed. Is there a variety? Are some activities for smaller groups or is everything scheduled for one big group? Are there activities scheduled throughout the day, evening, and on weekends? What plans are made for holidays? If you see something scheduled for the time of your visit, ask to observe that activity. If you are told it is not taking place, find out why. Take a look at the projects produced in arts and crafts sessions.

The idea is not to be a critic but to note the variety and appropriateness of the project for an adult person. A good activity program is carefully conceived and delivered with a focus on providing each resident with opportunities for personal enrichment, development, and motivation.

Activity programming can be one of the most important aspects of the nursing home service. The key question may not be so much how many staff but how active the residents are. Good programming will be structured around the capabilities of the residents and the involvement of others—volunteers, family members, and visitors. Still, this is another area where you will want to question staff-to-resident ratio. If the activity staff consists of one full-time and one part-time person to arrange activities for a hundred residents, they are understaffed!

Other Services

Another area of health care that is vital to the welfare and quality of life your relative will have in the nursing home is the food service. Food is not only nourishment for the body. The ritual of gathering for a meal or any occasion where food is served is a vital part of socialization.

Ask to see the kitchen, if possible during a meal. You do not need to take a "white-glove" inspection tour. Just look in and observe the situation. Are staff members properly dressed and groomed? Does the facility present a clean appearance? Does it seem well organized?

Ask for a menu for the week or month. Notice the variety in the meals. Ask what time meals are served. Ask about snacks. When are they available? What if a resident gets an attack of the "munchies" at three in the afternoon? Can he or she get a snack? have food in the room? go to a snack bar or vending machine? Do residents participate in selection of menu items perhaps through a food committee appointed by the resident council? Ask about special diets even if your relative is not currently on one. If possible, stay for lunch and observe the lunches served in the dining room. Certainly somewhere there should be a special meal—someone who needs the meal pureed, someone who cannot have milk products, etc. If you stay for lunch, make sure the meal you are served corresponds to the one listed on the menu.

Observe residents in the dining room. If possible, be in the dining room as they come in. See how they come together. Is there dialogue and conversation? Are some groups well established perhaps with members saving places for a latecomer? This is a good sign. It means these people at least have made some friends at the home and are building a social network. Notice or ask how many residents are fed in their rooms. Keep in mind that it is easier to serve residents in rooms than to get them into a dining room, but the opportunity to socialize in the dining room is very important.

There are other services you will need to ask about—laundry is a good example. Using your checklist, ask all the questions given, even if they do not seem applicable to your situation.

Finally, an intangible part of any resident's care plan is his or her emotional well-being. This will be difficult to judge because many of the people you will see when you visit a nursing home are very sick. Still, there are indicators. Ask if the home has a volunteer program and what sorts of functions that group provides. Ask if there is a support group for family members. Ask to meet a member of the resident council. Ask if there is a family council (a group made up of family members of residents who help in addressing problems and issues that may arise in the institution). Ask how the community is involved in the home. Do religious leaders come to the home? Do churches send vans or buses for those residents who may wish to attend services? Is there interaction between residents and younger people perhaps through a nearby school or community center?

Residents and Staff

Be sure to observe the people you see during your tour. Far too many caregivers visit a home and return to their relatives raving about the decor but with little information about the people they saw. Look at the residents. Talk to them. Pay attention to their sometimes unspoken messages. Are they dressed and active? Do they seem content and well cared for?

Be prepared to see some extremely sick and frail people. Be prepared to be approached by persons who are confused and disoriented. Nursing homes today have assumed a role of caring for people in the gravest stages of their illnesses. It is a testimony to family caregivers and community services that most older persons are able to live outside an institution all their lives. Keeping in mind that many of the residents you will see are in the final stages of their lives, direct your attention to the quality of care and attention to lifestyle being offered by the home.

Take a resident's hand in a gesture of greeting and notice the nails—manicured? clean? Notice the hair—again, is it clean? combed? When you stop to speak with a resident, take note of how the staff person who is guiding your tour deals with that encounter. Does the staff person attempt to speak for the resident? Does the staff person address the resident with the same respect he or she would give any other person? Does the staff person seem to know the resident and the resident's name? Does the resident appear to know the staff person?

In any nursing home you are going to see people sitting in the halls. Sometimes this is the resident's choice. He or she has come out of the room to observe the activity on the wing. Sometimes the person has been placed in the hall by a staff person and left there. If possible at the end of your tour, return to the areas where you started and see if the same people are still sitting with no sign of having moved or participated in any other activity. It is one thing if the resident is still sitting there and interacts freely with those who pass by. It is quite another if the person has been calling out or appears to be in need of attention he or she is not receiving.

It is also inevitable that you are going to see residents who are drowsy and listless on any given visit. But you should also see efforts being made to involve most residents in some way in the life going on around them even if their ability to participate may be severely limited by frailty and illness.

You also want to observe the staff as you move through the home. How are they dressed and groomed? Is there an air of pride and pleasantness in the way they perform their jobs? Do they greet you? Do they seem rushed and hassled? Why? Are they understaffed? Is it a particularly busy time of the day? If a call bell sounds or lights, how responsive are they? If someone sitting in the hall calls out to them, how responsive are they? Do they seem genuinely occupied by their job or are they visiting with each other?

Also take note of how staff react to the tour guide and you. One caregiver noted, "I toured three homes. In all three the tour guide was perfectly lovely, speaking to every resident, calling each by name. But in only one home did any other staff person speak to me or did the tour guide make any attempt to have me introduced to any other staff person. In fact, it was only in that home that the tour guide and staff people actually spoke to each other. In the other two homes there was not the slightest feeling that these staff people got along or had anything to do with each other."

One key problem in nursing homes (and other places where care is given to older persons) is something called *infantilizing.* This occurs when an adult speaks to another adult as if he or she were a child. "Are we ready for our bath, honey?" Or, "Let's put this bib on so you don't mess up that pretty little blouse." In many cases, infantilizing occurs without thought and without malice. Staff members do not even recognize they are doing it. Staff members who are genuinely fond of older persons may consistently refer to the residents as "Sweetie" and "Hon" without any recognition that there is anything wrong with that. This is often a sign of poor training rather than the fault of the staff person. However, while this behavior is not acceptable in most regions of the country, it is quite common in parts of the South and with some racial or ethnic groups. Cultural context is important in making judgments here.

When you meet a staff person, ask how long he or she has worked at the home. If it has not been long, ask where he or she worked before and why he or she changed jobs. If the staff person is a professional (registered nurse, administrator, social worker), ask where he or she received training and how long he or she has worked with older patients.

Besides residents and staff, note whether or not other people are in the home when you visit. You should see family members visiting relatives. You may see volunteers. Other persons from the community may have come in to present a program. Keep in mind that while you may find all this coming and going to be wearing, an older person who has been isolated for some time may find it to be exciting and stimulating.

Do not skip the tour. Many families never tour. Once they narrow their choices and satisfy themselves that the homes on the list are basically of equal quality, they sometimes try to abdicate the decision to the case manager or hospital social worker. "You choose; you know them better than I do."

But you are the person who knows your relative best. And in the absence of his or her ability to tour the home, you must be the eyes and ears of that person. Only by touring can you get a real impression of what life in this facility might be like. Only by talking with the staff, seeing the facility, and observing those already in residence can you decide if the home is right for your relative. It may be a beautiful and highly reputed facility, but if at all possible, you want to match the personality of your relative with that of the home.

When you tour, complete the entire checklist if you can. The more information you gather, the better able you will be to make an informed and successful choice. Do not rely on your memory. If you tour several homes, you may begin to confuse what you saw in one place with another.

When you tour, *take your time.* Notice everything, bring all your senses into play, and ask questions. The tour will probably be conducted by the administrator (if the home is small and/or locally owned) or admissions director. Whoever directs the tour should realize that you are under stress and pressure at this time and should be understanding and patient.

At the end of the guided tour, try to spend an additional half hour or so on your own. Walk through the home again. Stop to visit with a resident or two. Talk to some staff members you did not meet before. Talk to family members you see visiting. Ask them for positive comments as well as negatives. Take time to finish making any notes you need on your checklist. See if there was some area of the home you wanted to see but did not or some question you meant to ask but did not.

Along with all of this advice, you will need to accept some basic realities. The sad fact is that the choice of a facility most commonly is based on simple matters such as availability of a bed and location convenient for the caregiver. According to one survey, 51 percent of families in search of a home never toured one prior to placing their relative there. Only 24 percent based their choice on cleanliness, and even fewer gave the quality of staff, physical care, and programming as criteria they considered in their selection process. Perhaps the saddest statistic in this 1985 survey was that in only 10 percent of the cases did the resident play an active role in decision making.[2]

Another reality of nursing home life is that a nursing home is both a business and an institution designed to serve numbers of people rather than individuals just as a hospital is. It cannot replace home. It cannot offer each individual total autonomy. There are going to be limitations on movement and routine and personal privacy and freedom. With the increasing need for nursing homes to serve as acute care centers, there are going to be a lot of sick people, and that can be unsettling for the resident and for the visiting family. But regardless of age, health status, or place of residence, people share certain basic needs: a need to feel safe and secure, a need to belong, a need to feel personally worthwhile. And a well-run nursing home can meet those needs for those who require a level of long-term care they cannot get in the larger community.

[2]C. L. Johnson and L. A. Grant, *The Nursing Home in American Society* (Baltimore: The Johns Hopkins University Press, 1985), p. 63.

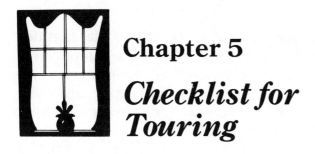

Chapter 5

Checklist for Touring

When you tour any home, take along the following checklist. It may not be possible to collect every bit of the information, but the list will help you to take an objective look at the home at a time when you are under stress and most likely reacting to circumstances in a subjective way. Fill in as much of the list as possible as you go. This will remind you to ask about issues and concerns you may otherwise forget. Do not be discouraged if you are leaving some items blank. The idea is to get as much data as you can so that it will be easier to make a decision. Do not be embarrassed about letting the tour guide see you taking notes. Nursing homes know these checklists exist—in fact, many nursing homes publish one of their own and encourage their use.

Some of the items on the list will be covered in your initial telephone contact with the home. Others will be best covered in your meeting with the home's admissions counselor or administrator. The rest are observations you will make as you walk through the home. If an item on the checklist is not relevant to your relative's situation, mark that item "NA" for "not applicable" and move on.

Regardless of whether this is an emergency tour or one in which you have the luxury of time, do not take shortcuts with the tour. Take the full time. Go through the entire checklist.

When you leave the nursing home, take a few minutes either as you sit in your car or as you have a cup of coffee at a nearby restaurant to review what you have seen. Do this immediately following the visit while details are fresh in your mind. Use this time to try to complete the Checklist Summary section. (See pages 75–77.)

If possible, tour a minimum of three homes—physically go to the home and take a tour. If you have more time and options available, tour more homes.

Nursing Home A: _____
                              (name of home)
  Tour conducted by: _____ Title: _____
Nursing Home B: _____
  Tour conducted by: _____ Title: _____
Nursing Home C: _____
  Tour conducted by: _____ Title: _____

First Impressions

_____ Atmosphere is warm, cheerful

_____ Personnel are courteous, helpful

_____ Staff seems enthusiastic, caring

_____ Residents seem well-cared for and content

_____ Residents are dressed in own clothing

_____ Resident rooms are personally decorated

_____ Room is available for private visits

_____ Written resident rights are offered and posted

_____ Residents, visitors, and volunteers offer praise for home

Physical Plant

____ Grounds are well-tended and entrance presents favorable impression

____ Home shows noticeable attempts to make environment more homelike and less institutional

____ Home appears clean and well-run

____ Home is free of unpleasant odor

____ Home is well-lighted

____ Public areas are decorated for residents, not visitors

____ Rooms are well-ventilated and temperature is comfortable

____ Hallways are well-lighted and wide enough for two wheelchairs to pass comfortably

____ Ramps outside allow easy access

____ Outside area is available for resident use

Safety

____ Home seems free of obstacles and hazards

____ Furnishings are appropriate for older persons with impairments

____ Toilets and bath/shower rooms have grab bars, rooms and baths have call bells, handrails in halls are all in place

____ Smoke detectors, sprinkler systems, emergency lighting are in place

____ Fire extinguishers are in place

____ Exits are clearly marked and unobstructed

____ Smoking and no smoking areas are clearly marked

_____ Directions for emergency evacuation are prominently displayed

Administration

_____ Administrator is available, courteous

_____ Administrator knows residents and staff by name

_____ Administrator is comfortable with residents

_____ Administrator is at the home most of every day

_____ Administrator appears to have good working relationship with staff

_____ Administrator shows concern and offers help

_____ Administrator offers freely any information requested

_____ Administrator offers incentive program and recognition opportunities to staff

Medical Services

_____ Resident's personal physician is welcome

_____ Home's staff physician is available to care for resident if chosen

_____ Physician is available on call at all times for medical emergencies

_____ Name and number of emergency physician are available to family

_____ Resident is seen by physician at a minimum every 30 days for three months and every 60–90 days thereafter

_____ Home has arrangements with nearby hospital for emergency transfers

_____ Home has plan with ambulance company for emergency transfers

_____ Family is notified prior to relocation

_____ Home offers dental care, eye care, and foot care (either as part of basic charge or at additional charge)

_____ Resident and/or family is involved in formulation of care plan

_____ Confidentiality is respected

Pharmaceutical Services

_____ Services are supervised by a qualified pharmacist

_____ Medications are properly stored and secured

_____ Resident can choose his or her own pharmacist

Nursing Services

_____ At least one RN or LPN is on duty on each shift

_____ At least one RN is on duty during the days, seven days a week

_____ Director of Nursing is RN

_____ Nurses (RN and LPN) and nursing assistants and orderlies regularly receive inservice training

_____ Staffing is adequate to numbers of residents

_____ Staff is willing to answer questions

_____ Number of residents is restrained

Rehabilitation and Therapy Services

_____ Therapists are either on staff or a contracted service that is a regular part of the home's care plan

_____ Therapies offered include:

    _____ physical

    _____ speech

    _____ occupational

    _____ recreational

_____ Therapies are included in basic rate

_____ Adequate space and equipment are available for offering therapy

_____ Social service counseling is available

Food Service

_____ Kitchen is clean and organized

_____ Waste is properly disposed of

_____ Kitchen staff is appropriately dressed, wearing hairnets

_____ Dietician is on staff

_____ Meal schedule is offered and displayed for residents

_____ Three meals are offered seven days a week

_____ Meals are served at normal hours

_____ Enough time is allowed for meals

_____ Nutritious snacks are available

_____ Food looks sufficient and appetizing

_____ Food is tasty and service is courteous

_____ Foods are served at proper temperatures

_____ Meal served matches menu

_____ Choice is offered if resident does not like particular food

_____ Special diets are observed

_____ Dining room is attractive and comfortable

_____ Dining room space is adequate for number of people served and for wheelchairs and walkers

_____ Atmosphere is pleasant, unhurried

_____ Residents needing help with eating are getting help

_____ Help with feeding is offered at no extra charge

Social Services and Recreational Therapy

_____ Trained social worker is on staff

_____ Ratio of social work staff to residents is workable

_____ Counseling and other social services are available to resident and family

_____ Activity calendar is offered and prominently displayed for residents

_____ Activity scheduled for time of your visit is taking place

_____ Residents are participating in activities

_____ Activities are varied to suit small or large groups and individual tastes

_____ Activities are realistic for older persons with mental and/ or physical impairments

_____ Activities include stimulus for the body, the mind, and the spirit

_____ Activities include outings away from the home for those who can participate

_____ Trained activities coordinator is on staff

_____ Ratio of activity staff to residents is adequate

_____ Suitable space for activities is available

_____ Suitable supplies are available

_____ Activities are offered for those confined to rooms or otherwise inactive

_____ Activities include events for evenings and weekends

_____ Home recognizes and respects individual religious preferences

_____ Residents participate in planning of activities

_____ Home offers

 _____ resident newsletter

 _____ resident council

 _____ family council

 _____ support group for families

 _____ resident "store"

 _____ chapel

_____ Home has volunteer program

_____ Home has active involvement from community in form of services and programs

Additional Services

_____ Personal laundry service is available

_____ Beauty/barber shop is available

_____ Snack bar is available

_____ Resident store is available

_____ Banking services are available

Resident Rooms

____ Room opens onto hallway

____ Room is reasonably near nurses' station

____ Room has window with a pleasing view

____ Room has no more than 4 beds adequately spaced

____ Resident has minimum of a bed, chair, reading light, closet, dresser, and bedside table

____ Closet and drawer space are adequate

____ Fresh drinking water is available

____ Call buttons are easily accessible

____ Home has plan for matching roommates

____ Room is large enough for both roommates to have walkers and/or wheelchairs

____ Curtain or screen is available for privacy in multiple-bed room

____ Toilet facilities are shared

   ____ with how many others

____ Resident is allowed to decorate

____ Current residents have decorated

____ Doors have nameplates of residents in that room

____ Resident is allowed a phone

____ Resident has easy access to public phone and privacy for use

____ Tour guide offers to show room on wing where resident would live

____ Tour guide introduces potential roommate

Baths and Shower Rooms

(Sometimes located away from patient rooms—ask to see!)

____ Facilities are conveniently located

____ Facilities are shared by how many residents

____ Safety features (grab bars and call bells) are in place and working

____ Resident receives bath/shower how often

Public Areas

____ Lounge areas for small gatherings for TV watching, cards, conversation, etc., are available on each floor or wing

____ Lounges are in use by residents

____ Telephone is available for resident use

____ Outdoor area is available to residents

____ Chapel or religious area is available

____ Private room for private family visits is available

____ No smoking areas are available

____ Isolation room and bath for resident with contagious disease are available

____ Visiting hours are convenient for residents and visitors

____ Areas are appropriately decorated with seasonal holiday decor or generally attractive decor

Residents

____ Residents are up, dressed, active

____ Residents seem reasonably content

_____ Residents move through home as if it is home

_____ Residents have made effort to personalize room or space

_____ Residents are comfortable talking to you

_____ Residents are easy with staff

_____ Residents know each other, talk, visit

_____ Residents appear clean, well-groomed

_____ Residents are not overmedicated

_____ Residents are participating in activities

_____ Residents speak and act freely

_____ Residents have family and friends visiting

_____ Residents have individual choices such as bedtime, freedom to move about the home, freedom to move if problems with roommate

Staff

_____ Staff members are attending residents, not gathered at nurses' station

_____ Staff ratio is reasonable for size of home

_____ Staff members interact well with one another, residents, and administrative staff

_____ Staff members receive regular inservice training

_____ Staff members appear to know residents

_____ Staff members are courteous, respectful, caring

_____ Staff members show interest in individuals

_____ Staff members treat residents with dignity and respect

_____ Staff members avoid childish nicknames ("Honey," "Sweetie")

_____ Staff members allow residents to speak for themselves when possible

_____ Staff members ask for resident preference when possible

_____ Staff members respect privacy (knock on room door before entering, close bed curtain before giving care, etc.)

_____ Staff members respond to calls for help in reasonable time

Family/Friends

_____ Visitors are encouraged

_____ Family and friends are in evidence while you tour

_____ Caregivers are willing to talk about home

_____ Families are offered services such as

    _____ counseling

    _____ care plan updates

    _____ support group

    _____ family counsel

    _____ family newsletter

Costs

_____ Home is affordable

_____ Monthly charges compare favorably with other homes

_____ Itemized list of basic services is offered in writing

_____ List of items not covered under monthly charge is available

_____ Additional charges are in keeping with same at other homes

_____ Refund is made for unused days paid in advance

_____ Admission contract is presented for consideration

_____ Home has clear procedures for transfer to hospital, for transfer from one room to another, for discharge from home offered

_____ Itemized bill is offered each month

_____ Deposit is required

_____ Payment plan is available

_____ Clear procedures are outlined for change in payment source (i.e., private pay to Medicaid)

_____ Adequate safeguards are in place for resident money and valuables

_____ Compensation is arranged for possessions lost or stolen

_____ Home encourages family to have attorney review contact and be present at signing

Questions to Ask in Meeting with Administrative Personnel

Discuss the following issues with the administrator, if possible, or address them to the person leading the tour:

1. Who owns the home? How long has it been owned by these persons? Are they a local group? If not, where are their headquarters? How many homes do they own?
2. What is the history of the home? How long has it been in business under the present owners? How has it grown? What is its present size (in terms of number of beds)?
3. What is the level of training for the administrative staff—administrator, director of nursing, director of social services? How long have these key people been in their jobs?

4. What is the daily or monthly rate? What does this specifically include? Can I have that in writing? What are the individual charges for other services? Can I have that in writing?
5. What procedures will the home follow if:
    - I or my relative has a complaint or concern
    - there is a medical emergency involving my relative
    - there is a change in the level of care needed by my relative
    - there is a change in payment source for my relative's care
    - there is a conflict between my relative and his or her roommate
    - there is a need for hospitalization beyond the normal period during which a room would be held for my relative
6. What is the staff turnover rate? Does the home "float" staff persons throughout the facility or leave the same people on the same wings and shifts? (Neither is necessarily good or bad by itself, but if your relative really needs stability as in the case of a person with Alzheimer's disease—you may wish to give preference to the staff that does not "float.")
7. What is the home's policy regarding responsibility for the disappearance of resident property?
8. What is the home's policy regarding the management of a resident's personal funds?
9. How does the home assign a room and roommate?
10. Can I have a copy of the home's admissions agreement or contract to study at home?

Before You Leave

Ask for copies of
- menus for the month
- activity schedule for the month
- names and titles of key staff persons
- name of staff physician or medical director
- list of resident rights
- list of basic and extra charges
- admissions agreement or contract

Checklist Summary for the First Visit

Did You Meet

____ administrator

____ director of nursing

____ director of activities programming

____ medical director*

____ social worker*

____ dietician*

____ therapist*

*Some of these people may not be permanently on staff or may not be essential for you to meet at this time.

Did You See and Note

____ nurses' station

____ pharmacy or medication storage area

____ therapy areas

____ isolation room for residents with contagious diseases

____ activity areas

____ lounges

____ chapel

____ dining room

____ kitchen

____ laundry

____ resident rooms (more than one if you could not be shown the actual room your relative would have)

_____ toilet facilities

_____ bathing/ shower facilities

_____ outdoor areas available to residents

_____ extra services areas such as resident store, beauty/barber shop, meeting rooms, counseling rooms, etc.

Did You Interact with and Observe

_____ residents in their rooms

_____ residents in the hallways and corridors

_____ residents during a meal

_____ residents during a scheduled activity

_____ residents during a therapy session

_____ residents being given a treatment

_____ nursing staff—both professional and assistants

_____ activity staff

_____ social services staff

_____ dining room staff

_____ maintenance and housekeeping staff

_____ administrative staff

_____ staff interacting with residents—nursing, programming, administrative

_____ staff interacting with staff

Did You Take Note of

_____ safety features such as fire doors, adequate lighting, lack of obstacles, handrails, and grab bars in appropriate places

_____ absence of unpleasant odors or cleaners used to cover same

_____ cleanliness of facility

_____ general condition of residents in terms of being dressed, being involved, being well-groomed and cared for

_____ attitude of administrator and other key personnel toward residents and toward other staff

_____ staff's familiarity and recognition of individuals rather than groups of residents

_____ residents interacting comfortably and naturally with one another and staff

_____ residents moving independently through the home

_____ resident rooms individualized

_____ staff observance and respect for privacy of resident by such actions as knocking before entering a resident's room and pulling divider curtain before administering treatments

_____ activities and meals that matched the schedule

_____ attitudes of affection, respect, and concern between residents and staff

_____ evidence of families and friends visiting

_____ evidence of involvement by others from the community such as clergypersons and volunteers

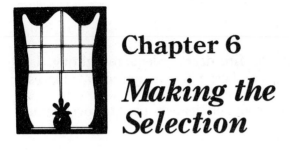

Chapter 6

Making the Selection

You are in the home stretch now, and the pressure to decide may be greater than ever for those of you who are dealing with an emergency placement. There are still three matters you must attend to before the final choice is made. Do not skip any of these steps. Each one is important to the final decision, and each is important for the adjustment process that will come later on for you and your relative.

1. Check the state survey records (available through the office of the ombudsperson) of the homes that most appeal to you.
2. Discuss your findings with your relative (if possible).
3. Make a second tour of the two homes you like best.

Checking the Survey

Most inspections are unannounced and are performed by a state-appointed team of professionals. Homes can be cited for violations that range from minor to major. You should know that much of the survey process concentrates on the physical plant and administrative management of the facility. You should also know that while survey reports are available for your consideration, you would do well to ask the ombudsperson or some other knowledgeable person to help you understand the report.

Some violations are relatively innocent and easily corrected. Example: A home may be cited for not having an extra chair in a resident's room. It may be that the chair was removed at the resident's request or that the chair had been moved on the particular morning of the inspection and by noon was back in its rightful place. This is a minor infraction of the regulations.

On the other hand, some violations are major, and their presence on a state survey report should act as a red flag to you regardless of what you thought you observed during the tour. In some cases a facility will be cited because it has consistently violated the same regulations with little or no attempt to remedy the problem. Citations for consistent understaffing or poor resident care are two infractions that should cause you to think carefully before choosing this particular home.

Again, rely on the ombudsperson to assist in your interpretation. For example, the ombudsperson may know that a home has recently been taken over by new owners who are making real efforts to correct problems and whose efforts you observed when you toured.

While you are talking with the ombudsperson, ask him or her about consumer complaints against the home from either residents, staff, or family members. If complaints consistently come in from staff, be forewarned. If the people who work there are upset with the facility, the result can be poor care. If concerns are raised by residents and family members, ask the nature of the complaints and how the home responded to them.

In the final analysis, a survey report may be helpful but should never be taken as the final word. There are too many variables—the best of homes may go through a crisis or transition period when standards are lowered. Also, survey procedures may vary widely and be tied to the availability and expertise of a survey team. Survey teams that are understaffed and overextended do exist. In addition, you need to allow for variations in the ability of the ombudsperson staff to know details about every home. Certainly, the survey check will add to your file of information, but in the long run your best source of information is the resident already living in the home and his or her family.

Reporting Back to Your Relative

There are few life events that are going to be any more difficult than telling your spouse, mother or father, or any other relative that the time has come for him or her to move into an institution. Over the course of caregiving, the chances are good that you have thought about the possibility more than once. But you dreaded the idea, and your natural instinct was to back away from any actual discussion of (much less planning for) the event.

In the long run, such tactics will probably result in more pain and damage to your relationship with this person than simple honesty might. One caregiving son who lived several hundred miles from his aging mother recalls the time he visited and recognized the possibility that on one of these visits he was going to be confronted with the need to choose a nursing home. His mother's physician had already raised the issue in a telephone conversation. So, on this visit, the son decided to see what was available in the area. He had never been in a nursing home and did not know what the process would be.

He could have just taken some time out of his visit and gone to the homes without saying anything to his mother, but he decided to tell her of his plan. She turned away in anger, and her eyes brimmed with tears. She refused to accompany him. In fact, she would not even speak to him. He almost decided not to go. But then he said, "I know this is painful and I hope we never reach the point where such care is necessary. But it's important to me to be prepared for any emergency. I live so far away and I want to know as much as I can before we have to do something under pressure. Maybe we'll never have to use what I find out today, but I have to see what's there . . . just in case."

There was no response, so he left.

A few hours later, he returned. He helped his mother prepare dinner in the kitchen. The conversation was spare and general. After a time, she asked quietly, "So, what did you find out?"

And with that unexpected beginning, he began to talk with his mother about nursing homes.

Not everyone will have such a positive experience. One caregiver said bluntly, "I lied. I said we needed to find a place until she could get better and I could bring her home." For some, the entire process will be met with recriminations ("How could you do this to me?"), anger ("I'd rather die first."), and all sorts of emotional baggage. But if the caregiver does not allow these tactics to take over the conversation, eventually the older person will have to deal with the realities of the situation.

Keep in mind that the way you and your relative deal with this topic will reflect the ways the two of you have handled any delicate subject in the past. If your mother's tactic has been avoidance or silence, you can expect the same thing when the subject of a nursing home is raised.

To help in dealing with your own emotions (so that you are better prepared to deal with those of your relative), begin by examining your feelings about nursing homes. Are you afraid of them? What is it you fear? Is there a basis for that fear? How sound is that basis? Perhaps in your view of nursing home life, your relative is going to be separated from friends and family and isolated in an institutional setting. But if you take the time to visit some homes, you will find that families are very much in evidence as visitors and even volunteers in good homes. You may see some residents leaving the home for outings with the family. And you will see opportunities for the development of new attachments within the home.

Some caregivers experience a feeling of failure. They feel that they have given up. One social worker told of the situation where a family insisted on taking the person home from the hospital when clearly the person could get better care in a professional setting. Still, the social worker agreed with the family's determination, because she knew they just needed to prove to themselves that they had done as much as possible. Within a week, they called to say they realized the nursing home was indeed the best caregiving decision they could make.

For other caregivers, the emotional impact is panic: panic that they have so little time to make the selection; panic that they will not make the right choice; panic that they are rushing into something. Spouses often express loneliness at the mere idea. Regardless of the mental and/or physical disabilities of the chronically ill person, the spouse feels an attachment and a loyalty and comradeship that are not lost even in caregiving

Many caregivers praise the idea of using the nursing home for respite care during those months and years when the person is being cared for by the family. Short-term stays help both the caregiver and the relative in that they show both that an adjustment can be made. If short-term respite stays can be in the facility the family would eventually choose in the event permanent placement became necessary, the older person may come to know other residents and staff even before he or she moves in permanently.

Another caregiving tool that can make acceptance easier for both parties is participation in adult daycare. Attending an adult daycare center gives the older person the experience of being cared for by a staff, of spending time in a communal setting, of taking part in activities and meals with a group of contemporaries. At the same time, the caregiver can see that his or her relative can accept change and can be well cared for by others.

How do you prepare your relative for the actual move? How do you include him or her in the preparations if that person is hospitalized or mentally impaired and unable to take part?

First, be honest. Too often, caregivers are overly enthusiastic in their zeal to make the home seem desirable. A nursing home is an institution—you know it and so does your relative. The patient is not going to be happy about the move in 99.999 percent of the cases. So present the facts in as positive yet honest a way as possible.

"Here's a brochure about the home. I think it has some nice features. For one thing it's right near my work so I'll be able to stop by often, maybe even come for lunch now and then. That's important to me. I met the lady who will be your roommate and she seemed nice. She used to shop at Dad's store and remembers seeing you there, too."

One nursing home admissions counselor prepares mini-photo albums of the facility for family members to take back and show the potential relative. The album takes the person on a tour of the home beginning with pictures of the exterior of the building and including pictures of the lobby, a resident's room, the dining room, therapy and activity sessions, and perhaps some special events that have taken place at the home. The snapshots are filled with people—staff and residents going about their life in the nursing home.

If the homes you visit do not have a brochure with pictures or snapshots you can borrow, consider taking some pictures yourself. A camera that makes instant pictures will serve you best in this case.

Discuss with your relative (if possible):

• Which facility would be the logical choice should a home be needed?
• What will be the pay source(s)?
• Is there a waiting list and can you place your relative's name on that list?
• What do you read and hear about the home?
• What was your impression when you toured the home?
• Do you know other families who have had someone living there? What have they said?
• What do the ombudsperson and the state survey have to report about the home?

This information is available for you at any time. You do not need to and should not wait until the eleventh hour to gather it.

No, the nursing home will never provide the kind of one-to-one attention the person can receive at home, but it can provide good care. And in some cases it can be not only the most loving, but also the most *appropriate* decision a caregiver can make with and for his or her relative.

Touring Again

You should make a second visit to a home for the same reason that you tour a house more than once before you purchase or rent it. You will want to pay attention to details you may have missed in the first visit and reassure yourself on any points about which you have doubts. The second visit should be slightly easier, because the place is now somewhat familiar and you are more sure of yourself.

On this second visit, you want to make certain you understand the following completely.

The Admissions Contract

Nursing homes may refer to this document by any one of many names: financial agreement, entrance contract, admissions agreement, etc. Whatever the terminology, your relative and/or you as the legal representative are being asked to sign a legally binding contract. Before this second visit, you will need to read the contract carefully, have it reviewed by your (or your relative's) attorney, and make arrangements to have that attorney present if there are serious questions about the document.

Basically, the contract should spell out:

• conditions under which the person is being taken in for care
  • services covered by the basic monthly rate
  • cost of those basic services
  • services that are *not* covered by the general rate
  • individual cost of each of those services
  • legal responsibilities of the home
  • legal responsibilities of the resident or guardian

The California Law Center on Long Term Care has published a paper on understanding nursing home agreements ("Consumer Guide to Nursing Home Admission Agreements"). The Law Center advises you to pay particular attention to and have your attorney review clauses that involve:

1. responsible party or guarantor
2. consent to treatment
3. Title XIX (Medicaid) eligibility
4. eviction or transfer
5. bedhold
6. resident's Bill of Rights
7. charges

8. notice of rate changes
9. security deposits
10. injury or loss
11. outside providers
12. medical records
13. photographs

If you or your relative do not have or cannot afford an attorney, ask the long-term care ombudsperson in your area to review the document with you before you sign it.

The Payment Plan
By the time you conclude your second visit, you should be clear about:

• how the nursing home care will be funded
• what sources are available to pay for that care
• how your relative becomes eligible to receive public assistance
• what is covered in the basic rate for each facility
• what is not covered and what these extra services cost
• how the resident will be billed
• what kind of refund policy the home has in the event the resident leaves the home or dies

Medical and Emergency Care
On your second visit, clarify any questions you have about the medical care your relative will receive at home. Is your relative's personal physician willing to continue to care for him or her in this home? How often will the physician visit? If you plan to have the home's physician provide care, has that physician met your relative, examined him or her, and consulted with the physician(s) who have provided care up to now?

What happens in the event of an emergency, or, barring an actual emergency, what happens if there is a marked change in the resident? Again, you want these policies in writing. If hospitalization is required, which hospital will the nursing home's medical director transfer the resident to? How long will the home hold the resident's room if he or she is hospitalized? How can you guarantee a longer hold? Does the administrator automatically notify you and the resident's personal physician in the event of emergency? immediately? before action is taken by staff?

Next, ask about the therapy your relative is to receive. What therapy has been ordered by the doctor? How long will the therapy continue? How will it be paid for?

Also ask about auxiliary medical issues and get policy statements about dental care, eye care, podiatry services, and pharmacy services. What are the home's policies regarding living wills and right-to-die actions? Ask what happens when a resident dies. What are the medical procedures and what are the *social* procedures? Does the home feel that death should be hushed up and handled as efficiently as possible without fanfare? Or does the home understand that older people know death is a part of life and seek to find ways to allow residents to grieve over the loss of a roommate or friend?

The Room and Roommate

On this second visit, if not on the first, you should certainly have the opportunity to see the actual room your relative would occupy and meet the roommate(s). Room locations and assignments will primarily depend upon the care needs of the resident as well as the availability of staff on any given wing and the availability of bed space within the home. Translation: In the good homes, which are almost always operating at capacity, you are not going to have much choice.

Walk into the room and check it out. Sit in the chair, try the light, open the dresser drawers and closet. Test the call bells by the bed and in the bathroom. Notice the pathway to the bathroom. Where is the nurses' station in relation to the room? Where is the shower/tub room? Where is the lounge?

When you meet the roommate, do not judge the person on your first impressions. He or she could be having a bad day and should be given the benefit of that possibility. On the other hand, if your relative is active, talkative, and ambulatory and the roommate spends his or her time in bed, cannot speak, and is heavily medicated, you will want to raise the possibility of another choice for your relative.

Transfer Policies

Not all transfers either within the institution or from the institution to someplace else are to the detriment of the resident. Sometimes, in fact, it is the resident and/or his or her family who instigate the change. There are three types of transfers:

1. transfers from one room to another within the home (this may include transferring from one wing or floor to another)
2. transfers from the nursing home to the hospital and possibly back again
3. transfers from this nursing home to another nursing home

Within each category of transfer are several possible reasons for the transfer. Transfers within the facility may result from a conflict between roommates. Or perhaps a change in the resident's condition requires a different level of care. For example, several homes today have special areas for their residents with Alzheimer's and related dementia. At first this resident may be able to function quite well on a floor with persons who have chronic physical limitations but who are mentally alert. In time, however, the level of supervision and care needed by the Alzheimer's resident may require a change of room to an area more specially geared to those needs.

Another type of transfer may take place within the home when someone with a private room moves into a shared room. This can happen when a person who has been private pay spends down and becomes eligible for Medicaid. Another instance where a room change may be desirable is the case of a married couple. By law, married couples have the right to share a room, but sometimes the paths of their individual illnesses will take them in directions where living apart is better than being together. The opposite problem exists when a married couple is separated upon admission because there are two available beds—one with a male roommate and one with a female roommate. In such a case, the couple may decide to take the available beds and wait for a room together.

Transfers from the nursing home to the hospital happen as a matter of course for all nursing homes. This is a procedure they see frequently and are used to dealing with. They usually have transfer arrangements worked out with an ambulance company and a nearby hospital—generally where the home's medical director is on staff. Your concern as caregiver is that you be notified of such a transfer, preferably before it takes place. You also need to be concerned about what happens to your relative's room and belongings while he or she is hospitalized and how long that room will be held for him or her.

Transfers from one institution to another are more rare than the other forms of transfer. Sometimes the resident and his or her family institute the change as in the case where the facility does not deliver the promised level of care, increases fees to a level that is unacceptable for the resident, or has changes in personnel that affect the resident's care or relationship with the facility.

Resident Rights

Somewhere in the home, a list of resident rights should be prominently displayed. You and/or the potential resident should be given a written copy of these rights when you visit. The key rights are listed in Appendix B on pages 161–164. Others may have been added to the list by the individual home or state.

Beyond a statement of rights, however, the home's staff should give clear indications that they value individual privacy. Such indications should be clearly visible if you look for them as you tour the home—staff interact with residents as responsible adults, not children; areas for private visits in person and by phone are provided; small quiet areas are as prevalent as large activity rooms and lounges; the pay phone is in an area where the resident who uses it has the dignity of privacy and quiet.

Routine and Care Plan

If your relative lives in this institution, he or she will develop a daily routine just as he or she had a routine at home. In this case, that routine or care plan will be developed by a team consisting of the medical and nursing, social services, and dietary staffs and hopefully the resident and you (if the resident agrees). The goal of this care plan should be to provide the individual with the greatest opportunity to live a meaningful and satisfying life and to improve his or her medical condition insofar as possible. The emphasis needs to be on quality of life.

If the home does not include the person and/or family member in the formulation of this care plan, that should be a red flag to you. How individually concerned can a place be that does not afford the resident or his or her spokesperson the opportunity for input? As a caregiver, you should be concerned with how much control over his or her own lifestyle the home is willing to allow the individual resident. Certainly you will understand that this is an institution and just like any institution (schools, hospitals, universities) has to have rules. What you seek is some clear indication that the home strives to keep those rules at a minimum and individuality at a premium.

When you sign the contract, you should make it known that you wish to participate actively in the development of a care plan for your relative and then make certain you are included.

Once you have toured all the homes on your list, take a moment to compare them with each other and with the goals you set for your relative when you began this search.

1. Compare basic and extra charges and services between the homes and rate homes according to 1, 2, and 3 (with 1 being the most desirable).
2. Compare the home's ability to serve you and your relative's needs in the following areas:
   - payment source
   - location
   - needed medical care
   - needed therapies
   - programming
   - food services
   - other services (dental, foot, ear, and eye care; counseling; services for family; etc.)

(In some areas, the homes may rate equally. Rate each home with a 1, 2, or 3 with 1 being the best again, then add up totals. Lowest total is the best.)

3. Based on your reactions (and those of your relative if he or she were able to tour) rate and add scores for:
   - administrative services
   - nursing care—professional
   - nursing care—aides and orderlies
   - programming
   - social services
   - other services (see above)
   - food service
   - housekeeping
   - maintenance

4. Based on your reactions and impressions, rate the home's efforts toward:
   - individualization of care
   - maintenance of independence and autonomy
   - fostering independence rather than dependence
   - deinstitutionalizing the home
   - programming that is creative and appropriate to residents
   - reaching out to and bringing community into the home
   - offering staff opportunities for training and incentives for providing superior care
   - showing concern for individual problems and concerns of residents and their families

   (This one will be difficult. You are going on one or possibly two visits to the home. You are going to have to rely in some part on your first impressions. This is another reason for remaining as objective as possible when you tour and may be an excellent reason to ask someone whose opinion you trust and who has no stake in the process to come with you when you tour.)

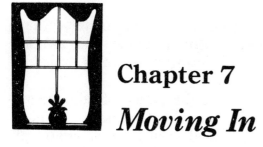

Chapter 7

Moving In

The nursing home has been chosen and your relative is about to make the move. There is a good possibility that the move will be made directly from the hospital to the nursing home without much time for preparation. Even if the move is being made from the older person's home in the community to the institution, the time for preparing the person for the move may be limited.

The hospital will make the arrangements for the transfer of the person from the hospital to the nursing home. The nursing home will tell you what the new resident needs to have in the way of clothing and personal effects for his or her residency in the home. A suggested list of what to pack (and what to leave at home) is given on pages 92-96.

If the home has a social worker on staff, that person is available to help both the new resident and the family adjust to this new lifestyle. If there is no social worker on staff, the administrator or admissions counselor can be helpful during the period of adjustment. You will need to draw on all your reserves of sensitivity and caring. Even if the person has agreed to the choice or seems incapable of understanding, you need to be aware that any change is going to be stressful.

The key is to involve the person in as much of the move as possible. This person is setting up a new home regardless of his or her incapacity or illness. In that light, you will want to protect the new resident's right to make decisions and maintain control over the new life as much as is possible. Even your attention to a detail such as time of check-in for the new resident may help ease the trauma of relocation. Nursing homes are busiest in the morning and around mealtimes, so the best time of day to move in is probably two to four o'clock in the afternoon.

Estimates vary on how long the period of adjustment lasts. Adjustment will depend on such factors as the new resident's state of mind, physical health, and emotional attitude at the time of admission. Some new residents adjust within a few days; others need several weeks. A small percentage of residents never adjust.

Choosing What to Bring

Once the home has been selected, start to involve your relative in decisions about what to pack. All clothing needs to be marked or have tags sewn in. Do that with the person, if possible. Do not forget to mark such items as dentures and eyeglasses. Help the person select some favorite framed photographs, pillows, artwork, and/or other personal items to take for decorating the room. If the nursing home gives its okay, plan to move a favorite rocker or chair into the room.

What Clothing Do You Take?

Plan to pack clothing that the person normally wears. If your mother has always dressed in slacks and blouses, do not go out and buy her a wardrobe of dresses or snapfront robes. On the other hand, if there is a very practical reason for a change in the normal style of dress (such as incontinence or impaired mobility), talk over the new style with your relative *before* you go out and buy the new wardrobe. If your father is most comfortable in dress slacks and shirts and he always wears a tie during the day, this is not the time to decide he would be more comfortable in something like a jogging suit, though it would be wise to choose dress slacks that can be washed. In general, the person should have enough clothing to change every day for a week without need of laundry service. If the person is incontinent, there may be a need to pack some extra clothing.

All clothing should be appropriate to the season and should be rotated with the change of seasons.

For men, pack:

- underwear
- outfits of the type he normally wears at home
- belts or suspenders
- pajamas
- laced sturdy shoes or slip-ons with backs (can be canvas, especially if the person is incontinent)
- socks
- slippers with firm, nonskid soles and backs
- washable cardigan sweaters
- flannel shirts
- a light jacket
- a warm coat
- gloves, hat, and handkerchiefs

For women, pack:

- underwear and hosiery (Girdles and pantyhose are difficult for most frail older women to manage even with help and should be left at home.)
- washable day clothes of the type she is used to wearing (slacks, dresses, skirts, and blouses)
- robes and sleepwear
- lace-up shoes
- slippers with backs
- washable cardigan sweaters
- purse
- coat
- hat, gloves

For the person who is very confused, add:

- clothing that is as simple as possible to manage—pull-on slacks or skirts, pullover tops, shoes with velcro closing rather than laces, etc.

For the bed patient, pack:

- hospital-type gowns
- washable robes
- slippers
- socks

Avoid any clothing that needs special attention such as handwashing or drycleaning.

What Else Do You Need to Mark and Pack?

Any of the following items the person normally uses needs to be marked and packed:

- toothbrush, toothpaste, denture supplies
- razors and/or electric razor, shaving cream, preshave and/or aftershave lotions
- cosmetics
- comb and brush
- talcum, face and body lotion
- manicure supplies—clippers, scissors, file
- shampoo
- tissues
- toilet kit for storing items
- shower cap

Aside from these personal care items and clothing, you will want to pack (if appropriate for your relative):

- smoking supplies
- hearing aid batteries
- stamps and stationery
- greeting cards
- carryall bags that fit onto walker or wheelchair
- a small change purse
- a clock and/or radio
- a small television
- one or two small easy-to-care-for plants
- some personal items that will help the person feel at home such as photographs, one or two small knicknacks, or a favorite afghan or quilt

• possibly a lock for the person's closet and/or nightstand drawer

And What about Furnishings?

You will have to check with the individual nursing home on this matter. In some cases, it may be possible for Dad to have his favorite recliner in his room or for Mom to bring her rocker. A small bookcase or other favorite piece might be possible, but do not count on it. Nursing home furnishings are frequently regulated by strict codes and standards. As much as the nursing home would like to support your efforts to personalize your relative's room, state regulations sometimes make such endeavors difficult.

Deciding What to Leave Behind

Do not bring anything of value—either monetary or sentimental value; leave it in a safe place at home and offer to bring it whenever the older person wishes to have it during your visits.

You also should not bring:

• medications or over-the-counter (OTC) drugs (the nursing home will handle the administration of prescription medications and any OTC drugs requested by the patient after first getting the patient's physician's okay)
• snack food unless you first okay it with the staff
• large sums of money (the resident should have some money available, and many homes will "bank" that money through the office so that the resident has access to it; but the resident should never have more than five dollars in his or her personal possession at any one time)

When possible, make plans with the person for those items that will not go with him or her to the nursing home. For example, not all clothing will go—some of it is inappropriate and there simply is not enough room for everything. Tell Mom that you have made arrangements to store things in your house or somewhere else, so if she needs a dressy dress for some special occasion, you can bring it.

Explain to your relative that items of real monetary or sentimental value could be lost, inadvertently taken by a confused resident, or even stolen. Do not automatically assume that the staff is to blame for such unfortunate losses. There is of necessity a lot of coming and going in a nursing home—delivery people, outside agency help, visitors, etc. Again, make plans to store such items safely and to have them available for those occasions when the person wants to see or use them. Example: Mom's diamond brooch could be kept in her safety deposit box.

Getting through the First Day

Ask if the nursing home offers an orientation program. Such a program or tour gives the potential resident a sense of confidence that he or she is not going to be totally unfamiliar with this new place of residence.

You should be getting the idea that the way to approach this period of adjustment is to give the older person as much control over his or her life as possible. Relocation of any sort is stressful for an older person. Relocation to a nursing home can often seem like the final surrender of personal autonomy and control. Your job as caregiver is to help the person maintain as much control and personal power as possible during these difficult days. Even if your relative is resistive and angry, plans need to be discussed openly and decisions and activities shared. Be open about what you plan to help him or her with. Handling the person's insurance and financial and legal affairs is one aspect of his or her care you may already have assumed and may continue to provide after the move to the nursing home.

Once you have decided what items will be moved from home, start to put together some items that will make the person feel more at home. If possible, take the person shopping. If not, plan a special housewarming basket filled with writing paper (if appropriate), paperback books, hobby supplies, pencils, pens, scotch tape, a small bulletin board (if allowed), a large-print calendar—anything that is appropriate to this individual. You might also have a telephone installed and/ or order daily delivery of the local newspaper.

A "nursing home shower" for a relative, in which friends and family are invited to come with shower gifts for the person and stay for refreshments is a positive approach. And this can be done any time—while the person is still in the hospital, on the day before the move, or a few days or even weeks following the move. (For ideas on what to give a nursing home resident, see pages 122-123).

You need to make some definitive plans for the first day at the home. This move is a major event in your relative's life and your life, and, as with any transition, the move will require adjustment. Your relative is going to have to adjust to life in a new environment—an unfamiliar setting where he or she does not yet know the routine. Your relative may experience feelings of loss—of being separated from the rest of the family, of being rejected or even unloved. He or she may deal with those feelings by becoming angry and resentful or by becoming passive in a way that indicates he or she has given up.

You are going to have to adjust to the change in your role as a caregiver and to the myriad of emotions that are accompanying this move. You may feel guilt at not being able to give the care needed. Having toured and made the choice, you may have second thoughts about whether or not you are doing the right thing. You may feel overwhelmed by the responsibility of it all, which may translate into some anger of your own.

Feelings

The key to dealing with your own and your relative's feelings about the actual move is to face them openly. Talk about them and encourage your relative to do the same. "Dad, I wish I could take you to live with me, but the doctor insists you need skilled care that cannot be given at home." Or, "Mom, I can see that you're really upset about this. It even seems like you're upset with me. I know it doesn't seem like it to you, but I really am trying to do the best I can for you."

Or even, "You're really upset about this, and so am I. Let's talk. I'll tell you why I'm upset if you'll tell me why you are."

Some of the factors that may come out of such a discussion include:

• fear there will be no privacy ("You're right. It won't be like home where you can do pretty much as you please. But there's privacy. You have your own space and if you don't want to be with anyone—even your roommate—you can pull the divider curtain.")

• fear staff will be abusive and uncaring ("I was worried about that too in light of some of the stories we've read and seen on TV. So I checked with the ombudsperson and she told me that this home has not had a single complaint filed against it in three years plus its state surveys have been excellent.")

• fear other residents will be demented or "senile" ("I met some of the residents when I toured and I saw others participating in activities. I'm not going to kid you, there were some confused people there. But on the wing where you will be, the residents were more like you. In fact, that's the policy of the home—to group people of like abilities together.")

• fear of being forgotten ("Forgotten by whom? the staff? They really seem to care, and how could it be an act? They have tours going through all the time. Or are you afraid we'll forget you? I've already told you that I'll be by for sure every Tuesday and Thursday and we still plan to have you join us for Sunday dinner, just like always. In fact, maybe sometimes we'll join you for Sunday dinner there at the home.")

• fear of never being able to leave the home even for an outing ("There are residents at the home who are pretty much bedbound, but you're not one of them. I brought you the listing of activities for this month and look, there are at least two outings planned. Not only that, but I spoke with your clergyman and he said there is a special van that picks up residents from the home and brings them to services.")

• fear that life there will be boring and dull ("Only if that's your choice. If you choose to sit in your room or in the lounge staring at a TV set all the time, they may just let you do it. But there is plenty to do if you choose to get involved. In fact, I want us to talk about those activities you want to participate in once you get there, so that my visits won't interfere with something you want to do at the home.")

• fear of losing all control and individual freedom ("I brought you a copy of this document they call 'The Resident's Rights'—this is the law. Such things as your right to information, to personal privacy, to personal freedom, to be treated with respect, to complain without fear of retribution are protected by not only the state but the federal government.")

At this point you may need to note to your relative that with rights come responsibilities. He or she has a responsibility to respect the rights of the other residents in the home and to treat other residents as well as the staff with the same courtesy and respect he or she expects to receive.

Certainly not every potential resident experiences or expresses these fears. Your relative's historical approach to stress and life in general should be a good indication as to how he or she will respond to the stress of relocation to a nursing home. In one instance, an eighty-year-old widow's friends were shocked and dismayed when they heard she was moving to a nursing home. They accused the woman's children of not caring and of putting her away. But when they spoke to the woman, they found that she had made her own decision. "It will happen sometime soon," she told them. "Every time I have to go back to the hospital there's a greater chance so I decided to make the move now while there's a bed available at this home that I like."

Actions

Some homes will welcome your staying all day with the new resident. Perhaps a better arrangement, though, would be to help the person move in (early afternoon is a good time) and get his or her initial bearings, then turn the person over to the expert care staff (this means leave), come back later in the day perhaps to have dinner with your relative, and find out how the afternoon went.

Stay with him or her until bedtime and then go home. At night, reality begins to set in, and it can be a frightening reality. Your presence can be a real comfort during that first evening until the person has settled down and gone to sleep. This "first night phenomenon" may be a matter you wish to discuss with the staff when you tour the home. What special plans do they make for comforting new residents during that first night? Their answer could give you a good indication of the level of concern and care that will be offered in this home. Call the next morning to see how things went during the night and let your relative know when to expect your next visit.

If you are a long-distance caregiver and have come into town to help the person relocate, do not spend all your time with your relative. That isn't healthy for either you or your relative. Instead, use the time to clear up whatever loose ends may exist following the relocation.

One positive step that you can take for both you and your relative is to find someone to whom you can delegate the responsibility for staying in touch with your relative and notifying you of problems. In many communities there are case managers who will oversee the care of an older client. To find out if a case manager is available in your relative's community, look in the Yellow Pages under Social Workers or Social Service Agencies, or call your local Office on Aging or ombudsperson's office. Many states have programs that offer volunteer guardians for persons in nursing homes. You may wish to hire a social worker (not one who works for the home) to check on your relative on a regular basis. A former neighbor or good friend may be willing to assume this responsibility. Whomever you recruit, take the person with you to visit your relative and explain what his or her interaction will be.

If the person moving to the home is extremely confused, adjustment will be different. Confused persons are often filled with anxiety and may cling to you whenever you appear. You are familiar to the person, even though he or she may no longer recall that you are a daughter or spouse. You can help the person adjust by always visiting at the same time of day so that your visit can be anticipated. Also, it is a good idea to let the staff know your plans so that they can reassure the person. On the days you cannot visit, call, and call between visits if you think it is necessary.

Begin immediately to get to know the staff persons who will give care to your relative—especially the nursing assistants. Let your relative see that you like and trust these people. Talk to the social worker and nursing staff about ways you can help the person adjust. They have seen many confused residents, and they may have some very good advice for you.

If the new resident is extremely ill and perhaps in bed most of the time, you will want to give special attention to his or her comfort within the room. Again, get to know the staff and help the person to know them as well. If possible when you visit, take the person out into the home using a wheelchair. If there is the possibility of an improvement through therapy, show that you believe in that possibility by encouraging and assisting the person with his or her exercises. (Ask for instructions before you try this.) Keep in mind that for the very ill resident, his or her space in this room is pretty much the world. Try to make that world as pleasant as possible.

Your involvement in this adjustment process is very important and cannot be overstated. However, as you read before, it is also important that you not set a pattern in these first days that you will find difficult to live up to after a time. Decide now on a visiting schedule you can live with for a long time to come . . . once a day, three times a week, whatever you find manageable. Spouses are particularly guilty of spending too much time with their loved one in the nursing home in the first weeks. When the spouse is there, the resident has no need to get out and take part in activities or in meeting other people. Later, when the spouse has to cut back on visits, the adjustment is twice as difficult.

Getting to Know the Personnel

When someone moves into a nursing home, that person becomes a resident in a new place with new neighbors and new people providing services. It will take time to adjust—from all sides. The staff will need to adjust to your relative at the same time he or she and you are adjusting to them.

You have been so busy choosing the home, adjusting to the idea, getting the move made, and helping your relative get used to the change that you may not have given much thought to the individuals who will be caring for your relative for the next several months and possibly for the rest of his or her life.

The staff of a long-term care facility is made up of a diverse group of people—the larger the institution, the more staff there will be. Basic care and services are provided by persons within the facility working in various departments and under the supervision of the facility's administrator. Other services may be contracted from outside the home, and these persons may not be permanent members of the health team within the home. Whether services are given by in-house or contracted personnel, the basic titles and responsibilities remain the same.

Nursing Assistant

These men and women will provide the great majority of services your relative will receive. They bathe and feed residents, assist with personal care such as shaving and dressing, accompany residents to and from activities and therapies, and generally oversee the daily routines of your relative and the other residents of the home. In addition to those defined duties, it is quite possible that these are the persons who will be there (or not) to hold your relative's hand when he or she is upset or lonely, to reassure, to spot changes in health or mental status, to encourage participation, to listen, and to understand.

Given this range of responsibility, you may be surprised to learn that training for this position is usually provided on the spot. Fortunately for both the nursing assistants and the residents they serve, the nursing home reform act of 1987 mandates that there must be a training program for these persons in any home certified to receive any federal funds such as Medicare and/or Medicaid.

Activity Coordinator

This person has possibly the second most important job in the basic care of your relative. He or she is responsible for planning the daily routine of activities and programs that will enhance life for your relative in the nursing home. While some activity coordinators are highly trained in their field, many are hired because they have some qualifications for doing arts and crafts with little attention paid to their ability to work with frail and impaired older persons.

In spite of the lack of availability of higher-level training for their positions, both nursing assistants and activity coordinators consistently are dedicated, caring individuals who work hard to provide good care and quality programming for residents.

Licensed Practical Nurse (LPN or LVN)

Licensed nurses have had one year of training in nursing and have passed state licensing examinations. LPNs may administer medications and perform some nursing treatments. In many homes, an LPN may be the nurse in charge of the wing or floor, particularly during the night shift. Today, LPNs perform many of the nursing services that once were performed exclusively by RNs.

Registered Nurse (RN)

This person is also licensed, but he or she has had two or more years of training before passing the licensing examination. The RN in the nursing home is the person who assesses the resident's needs and oversees the development of a care plan for that resident. He or she may administer medications, perform treatments that require skilled nursing, and also function in a supervisory position.

Charge Nurse

The charge nurse—hopefully an RN—is in charge of the wing or floor on any given shift. He or she functions as the supervisor for other RNs, LPNs, and nursing assistants on that wing/floor for that shift.

Director of Nursing

The director of nursing is an RN responsible for overseeing all nursing personnel in the home as well as supervising the implementation of care for all residents. This person works closely with the administrator and other senior staff and is instrumental in setting the overall philosophy for the facility.

Medical Director

This is a physician who has been retained by the facility to direct policy for medical care in this home. If a resident does not have a personal physician when he or she enters the home, the Medical Director will assume responsibility for that person's medical care during his or her stay in the facility.

Administrator

The administrator is responsible for supervising the business and organizational operation of the facility. He or she hires (and fires) staff, establishes policy, sets standards, oversees the physical plant, maintains the facility, balances the budget, oversees the business administration of the home, and generally acts as chief troubleshooter and policymaker for the home.

Not enough attention is given to the way in which this person performs his or her job. Because it is a nursing home, the focus is often on the medical staff. But the administrator is the head of this healthcare pyramid. If the home you choose is managed by an administrator who does not see himself or herself as responsible for maintaining the *health* (as opposed to the illness) of an individual, you and your relative could be in trouble.

Board of Directors or Owners

You may never meet any of these people. They are the financing source and/or the policymakers for this facility. Their philosophy will be reflected through the administrator and passed through him or her to the rest of the staff. If this group is a local one, you may well see them at the home taking an active role in its administration. If, on the other hand, the home is owned by a national organization or corporate chain, you may never see these men and women. Still, their idea of how care can be given with maximum efficiency and minimal cost will affect you and your relative in a very personal way.

Records and Business Department

This is the office where medical records are kept and the business of paying for services is transacted—bills are prepared, personal funds are handled, supplies are ordered, etc.

Supportive Services

No home could operate without the services of persons who handle the upkeep, housekeeping, and general operation of the home. These persons may be employed in departments of food service, housekeeping, laundry service, and/or maintenance. Their jobs are frequently low-paying, unskilled positions, and yet they are members of the care team as surely as any other employee of the home.

In addition to these in-house staff members, other staff may either be permanent staff members or come into the home on a regular, part-time basis. These persons include:

Therapists

Therapy, as you have seen, plays an intricate role in the quality of life a person may enjoy in any long-term care facility. The men or women who provide these restorative services are trained in their fields and include physical therapists, occupational therapists, speech therapists, and recreational therapists. Their responsibility is to work with the nursing staff to implement a care plan for each resident while providing a program of activities that will enhance the lives of all residents.

Social Worker

In a way, the social worker is a member of both the nursing and therapy staff. He or she is a vital link in the chain of good care in a long-term facility, and you may want to question why such a person is not a permanent member of the home's staff if he or she is not. Social workers are trained professionals. Their duties in the long-term care facility include helping residents, families, and other staff understand and accept the person's illness, impairments, care plan, and needs; handling resident and family concerns and complaints; encouraging maximum participation of the resident in the life of the home; and providing opportunities for counseling and support to both the resident and the family.

Dietician

The entire food service of any facility may be a contracted service with the head of that agency hiring his or her own kitchen and serving help. A dietician is responsible for planning nutritious and attractive meals and snacks for residents and for working with other staff to meet individual needs pertaining to food service and nutrition. For example, if a person needs a special diet or food prepared in a special way, it is the responsibility of the dietician and food service to see that these requirements are met.

Ancillary Medical Personnel

Podiatrists, dentists, ophthalmologists, and pharmacists are all important links in both medical care and quality of life for your relative. Just because a woman rarely leaves her room and only walks occasionally is no excuse for ignoring basic foot care and properly fitted shoes. Just because a man is 92 does not mean he should not have the right to properly fitted dentures that allow him the luxury of a varied diet. And just because a resident has severe glaucoma that has already taken the sight of one eye is no reason not to attend to the resident's remaining sight in a vigorous and aggressive manner. Certainly the pharmacist is going to be an important link to care for any resident. He or she is responsible for the safekeeping and proper delivery of prescribed medications for each resident. While medications are administered to residents by nursing staff, it is the pharmacist who sets the model for the way that facet of medical care is delivered.

Community Services and Volunteers

Many homes have regular services provided by members of the community. For example, almost any home worth its reputation as a long-term care center will offer religious services for all denominations. Clergypersons should be on call for the home, and the home should have an active relationship with several clergypersons from the surrounding community.

More and more homes are offering residents the option of an in-house beauty and barber shop. Several homes have stores where residents can go shopping for small necessities and snacks. Some homes have snack bars and/or soda shops, and a few even offer restaurants.

In a growing number of long-term care facilities, the administrative staff is beginning to see the need for and advantages of opening the home to more interaction with the surrounding community. To this end, many homes have actively pursued volunteers from the neighborhood and linked up with other institutions within the community such as schools and service clubs to offer programming in the home. Some homes have set up a daycare center for children of employees in the home. This affords many opportunities for intergenerational activities between residents and the children, plus it personalizes staff members for the residents.

Family, Friends, and Other Residents

Yes, you are part of what the American Health Care Association calls a "circle of care" for anyone who resides in a long-term care institution. Your input and interaction with the resident, other residents, and the staff can make the difference between an experience that is positive and one in which the resident is miserable and isolated. Since half of all persons who live in nursing homes have few or no visitors, you can make a difference for not only your relative but other residents as well.

Ombudsperson

While this person is not actually on the staff of any individual home, he or she is a vital member of the care team. The position is federally mandated, with the person appointed by the state, and was created through the Older Americans Act. The ombudsperson serves as advocate and mediator for all nursing home residents and their families within a particular area.

P·A·R·T
TWO

•

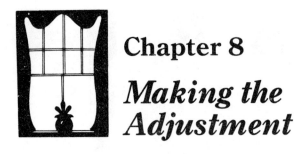

Chapter 8

Making the Adjustment

Your responsibilities as a caregiver change once the person moves to a nursing home. Now that the hands-on, day-to-day care is being provided by the institution, you have the opportunity to take on new roles as advocate and guardian for the resident's interests. You also have the opportunity to continue to offer care in very special ways, such as by doing the person's laundry, by arranging outings for the resident, and by being available to listen and share in ways you may not have had time for before.

Helping the Person Adjust to the New Home

In the first weeks of residency in a nursing home, your best friend may turn out to be the home's social worker. It is his or her job to assist both the resident and the family in this delicate time. What is important for the new resident are the same things that would be important for anyone placed in a new and strange situation. Did you ever have to transfer schools, start a new job, or move to a new neighborhood? What was important? to be accepted, wanted, safe and secure? to feel a sense of belonging, of being significant, of making an impact or contribution? The same things are of importance to the new nursing home resident.

Dr. Michael Hunt, architect and professor at the School of Family Resources and Consumer Sciences at the University of Wisconsin-Madison, notes that "confidence in way-finding [finding one's way around the facility] can influence whether residents will come out of their rooms, engage in activities and meet new friends. These behaviors indicate the elderly person's healthy adjustment to a new setting."[1]

Your goal is to make life in the nursing home as normal as possible. To that end, you may want to keep the following tips in mind:

- Set a pattern for visiting (see page 118).
- Keep your promises. If you say you are coming at a particular time, be there. If you say you will call, call. If you say you will take the person out for lunch, be definite about when.
- When you visit, conduct yourself as if you were visiting the person in his or her home. If possible, let the person take you out into the home or into the dining room for lunch.
- Include the person's roommate in some of your visits. This helps to foster a better relationship between these two people and also allows you to gauge how things are going.
- Bring children, grandchildren, former neighbors, and/ or friends with you when you visit if possible.
- Take the person out whenever feasible.
- If the home allows it, bring in the family pet for a visit.
- Find ways to involve the community system the person was active in—his or her religious home, clubs, or charities. For example, if Mom once did volunteer work for the Red Cross, might she still be able to help out by stuffing envelopes or folding flyers? Can the clergyperson visit? Can the new resident still go out to attend his or her own church or synagogue?
- Encourage involvement in the home's activities. Make it clear that you want to check the best time for your visit against the planned program of activities in the home. But be realistic. If your relative was not much of a "joiner" or social person before, it is not likely this person will suddenly

---

[1]M. Hunt, "Reducing Relocation Stress," *Parent Care*, Vol. 3, No. 2 (January/ February, 1988), p. 5.

blossom into one now. Respect the individual's right to ease into life in the nursing home in his or her own way.

• Continue to involve the person in the life of the family by seeking his or her input and advise on family matters. If there is a family event coming up such as a wedding, birth, or reunion, find some way to involve the person in the plans.

• Listen.

• Touch.

Assessing Adjustment

How these goals are achieved will depend in large part on the nursing home staff, you, and the rest of the resident's support system, as well as the resident. Praise any effort by the staff to allow the resident to take part in decision making. Meet with other members of the family and outline a plan for support during these first difficult weeks—perhaps hold this meeting with the nursing home's social worker, who can advise the family on what is too little help and what is too much.

The roommate can also be an ally. While adjustment between these two people will not be automatic, with time a real friendship may develop. The dynamics at work here are awesomely against getting along. The roommate may have become very attached to his or her former roommate and resent the loss. Your relative may be unused to living in such a confined space and having to share that space with someone else. Territorial rights have to be negotiated: If both roommates have wheelchairs, is there enough space for moving around easily? What if the bathroom's location requires one roommate to cross another roommate's space? And then there is noise: Roommates can resent having to cope with each other's television habits, sleep habits, wake-up habits, and visitors. Something as simple as whether the shade should be pulled or left open can be fodder for a major disagreement.

"The search for a familial community within a nursing home demands persistence," according to Joan Retsinas.[2]

[2]J. Retsinas, *It's Okay, Mom: The Nursing Home from a Sociological Perspective* (New York: The Tiresias Press, Inc., 1986), p. 57.

There are all sorts of barriers. The design of the home itself may be a barrier: Heavy fire doors and elevators reserved for use by staff may inhibit free movement. Also, the residents themselves may pull back. The idea of impending death in the nursing home may cause many to resist forming attachments of any sort.

There are a number of indicators you can look for in assessing the resident's adjustment. For example, in the dining room, residents will usually settle at one table, in fact in one particular place at that table. This becomes that resident's established place—the importance, again, of territory. From here, he or she can be as social or private as desired. The same thing goes for the lounge area and in the activity programs. When you see your relative beginning to assert himself or herself in terms of territory, you can know that adjustment has begun.

Another factor in the adjustment process is mobility. Mobility does not simply mean the freedom to move through the home. It can mean something as basic as the ability to move from one's bed to a wheelchair without help, to be able to walk down a corridor with the help of a walker or handrails instead of always having to call an assistant. It can mean being able to feed oneself, or relearn such basic grooming skills as shaving or tying shoes.

Incorporating therapy into a new resident's plan of care can make the period of adjustment easier. Therapy (physical, occupational, speech, and/or counseling) provides a meaningful activity where the focus is on wellness rather than sickness. Nancy Fox notes that ". . . Section four of the Older Americans Act calls for 'full restorative services for those who require institutionalization' . . . . This is a nursing home, a convalescent center. Remind yourself again that this is not a hotel."[3]

Rehabilitation and care go well beyond basic medical services and formal therapies. There are also the therapy elements that come through in the very environment—the

---

[3]N. Fox, *You, Your Parent, and the Nursing Home* (Buffalo: Prometheus Books, 1986), p. 104.

paint on the walls, the choice of lighting, the choice of artwork, the decor of individual rooms. Opportunities for activity as well as opportunities for privacy are a part of therapy. Being encouraged to pursue former life interests can be therapeutic. Meeting a volunteer or group from the community can be therapy. Holding a staff person's baby or petting the family dog can be therapy. Having one's hair done can be therapy. For a man, going to the barber shop where a male barber cuts and shaves and gossips and talks about politics and ball scores can be therapy.

Families can assist the resident in the pursuit of increased independence in a number of ways:

• recognize that if the person is moody and unresponsive, he or she may be using the only available defenses in order to adjust
• know the program of treatment for the resident
• find out how you can help when you visit
• arrange to visit at a time when you can observe and perhaps assist in therapies and programs designed to rehabilitate the resident
• encourage and assist the resident to move around his or her room and the rest of the facility; make *movement* a purposeful part of the visit, if possible.

You will want to temper your involvement with respect for the resident's wishes. Sometimes a family member's presence is embarrassing or distracting to the resident. Sometimes families try to help too much and hinder the progress of the patient. And sometimes family members are unable to disguise their impatience or distress at the clumsiness and/or slowness of the patient.

You will quickly learn that some residents of nursing homes have no immediate family or caregivers in town. In fact, this lack of a community support system may be the reason the person came to live in the nursing home. Some of you may be long-distance caregivers who will not be able to visit your relative on a regular and frequent basis. You need to understand the magnitude of what all residents are facing—even those who have devoted family and visitors.

When you are not around, these older persons are being asked to live among people who have never known them, who do not know them now, and who may express little interest in getting to know them beyond what their basic care needs may be.

Your goal is to assist this person you love in making a successful adjustment to a new lifestyle by helping him or her to find meaning and purpose in that life. At no time should the resident feel he or she is being forced to accept routine or that he or she is being pitied.

Finally, keep in mind that people who make it to old age have already survived an incredible number of life's hard times and tragedies. They made it this far on their ability to adapt and cope, so do not sell them short now.

Making Life Easier

Recognize and respect the older person's right to some privacy even when he or she is surrounded by people. Often you may see residents in nursing homes, perhaps even your own relative, sitting quietly in their rooms or alone in a quiet area of the home. Do not necessarily be alarmed at this.

Privacy is as necessary to good health as socialization is.

Privacy gives us a chance to take a respite from all the hustle and bustle of what is going on around us. The nursing home is a busy, often noisy place.

Privacy also gives a person the opportunity to just be himself or herself for a while without having to worry about the social graces or keeping up conversation or being polite. When a person is denied privacy over too great a period of time, you may see some adverse results. The person may withdraw and isolate himself or herself. The person may become irritable and even angry. Complaints of being tired or apathetic may be symptoms of a need for some respite and privacy.

How can you guarantee privacy for your relative? Help him or her search out little-used and quiet spaces in the nursing home. Perhaps there is a reading room or library. Perhaps there is a small alcove without much traffic. Or perhaps he or she can simply be in the room and draw the divider curtain. Wherever you find these opportunities, encourage your relative to make use of them when he or she feels the need to get away for a short while. Especially if your relative has always been a rather quiet person, you will want to show him or her that you understand the need to find a place to escape to for a short time. Inform the staff of this need, and enlist their aid in making these "mental getaways" possible.

When you visit, talk honestly with your relative and try to elicit his or her feelings: "I know how you must miss being at home." Don't say, "You're really better off here." Say, "We miss you and so does your neighbor." Don't say, "You should be grateful for all the time we've spent finding this place and getting you settled here."

Also, talk about the family and other matters of interest to the resident in the same way you would if that person were at home. Make him or her feel a part of the world beyond the nursing home. You may encounter some unusual behavior during this time of adjustment—confusion, disorientation, anxiety, and anger—where there was none before. Do not let these new reactions deter you from maintaining your communication with your relative. He or she may be grieving—this relocation can be considered a major loss, and grief is normal and even healthy.

Watch for signs of anger directed at the staff—particularly at the nursing assistants. Your relative may be angry at the family but take it out on these strangers.

Encourage the person to participate actively in the life of the home. When you visit, talk about what is going on in the resident's life. The two of you should have many new things to talk about. If your relative is confused and perhaps unable to recall what he or she did that day or the day before, ask the staff before you enter the room to fill you in. Then bring those things up. "Lisa told me you made a real breakthrough in physical therapy this morning." Or, "Can you tell me about the musical program they had last night?"

Surprise your relative from time to time with special treats—not just food but perhaps a trip to the home's beauty/barber shop or a shopping jaunt to the home's store to choose a birthday present for a favorite grandchild. Bring in photographs and encourage the resident to share them with staff members. In these early weeks, one of the things you can do to make life more pleasant is to allow the staff to get to know your relative beyond being the "woman in 306." And it goes both ways. By pulling the staff into your relative's life, you pull yourself and your relative into the staff person's life. You learn about the people who are providing care in a personal way that makes them more than just employees.

In their publication *Parent Care*, the Gerontology Center at the University of Kansas cites the following "4 R's" of adjusting to a nursing home as attributed to Bernard Reisman, Director of the Hornstein Program in Jewish Communal Service, Brandeis University:

- *Reassurance*—family and friends spend significant time there during the first days and weeks telling the resident how much they recognize and appreciate the adjustment he or she is making to this new and difficult situation
- *Routes*—family members can do their best work in these early days by helping the new resident to find the best routes for moving about the home and finding his or her way safely and with confidence
- *Routines*—the repetition of basic daily routines helps the patient to establish a pattern of life that becomes comfortable and reassuring in and of itself
- *Relationships*—as discussed above, the family can be a link to building friendships between the new resident and other residents as well as staff members

Making Visits Count

The time you spend with your relative in his or her new place of residence is an important facet of this person's new lifestyle. Making visits something both you and your relative anticipate with pleasure is going to take some work—mostly on your part. Keys to good visits include:

- knowing when and how often to visit
- knowing what to talk about and when not to talk
- knowing what to do and not to do while visiting

• knowing how best to approach special occasions such as birthdays, family events, and holidays

As far as the nursing home staff is concerned, you can make their lives easier if you:

• observe visiting hours whenever possible (although the 1987 nursing home reform act gives family members the right to be in the home with their relative any time)
• do not bring in food or such things as medications or smoking materials unless you first check with the nursing staff
• call rather than visit in person if you are not feeling well yourself
• confine your visit to normal visiting areas of the home— lounges, lobbies, the resident's room
• do not try to administer care yourself (help your relative to the bathroom or administer medications) unless you first check with the nursing staff
• bring any problems to the staff's attention as soon as possible
• do not stay past the time the resident can tolerate the activity and do not leave babies and children who are visiting unattended
• limit telephone contact during the morning hours when the nursing home is at its busiest
• let staff know in advance if you plan to take the resident on an outing so they have time to get the resident dressed and ready and medication prepared as needed
• include other residents in your visits, especially those who do not have many visitors

The Visit—a Part of the Care Plan. What goes on when you visit can be an integral part of your relative's care. If handled properly, a visit can be as productive a therapy as any planned program the facility may be able to offer. Understand that you will probably never visit often enough to suit your relative. On top of that, confusion and mental impairment may cause your relative to forget your visit almost as soon as you leave the building. But the staff knows how often you are there. They see you and the care you bring with you and that helps them to look at your relative in a more positive light.

As for the family unit itself, some caregivers have found that their relationship with their relative has actually improved following the nursing home placement. On the other hand, many nursing home staff members note that overwhelming guilt sometimes causes caregivers to visit too often. In so doing, they effectively eliminate the need for the resident to adjust to and participate in nursing home life. A feeling that you have abandoned Mom or Dad can urge you to spend more time in visiting than is healthy for either you or your relative. Many caregivers visit every day, call every day, and relay the smallest matters to nursing home staff in their zeal to prove that they have not deserted their loved one. The nursing home staff understands that your relative needs the level of care offered by their facility. You don't have to prove yourself to them. Normal interaction between you and your loved one on a regular basis is what is called for.

The Visit—the Difference between Success and Disappointment. In the hospital setting, visitors come to the room, chat awhile, and leave. Often they bring gifts. The conversation centers on the health of the person and the progress of his or her hospitalization. They always know the number of times they visit will be finite. No one stays in a hospital forever. In the nursing facility, many visitors conduct the visit as if they were coming to a hospital. And this is a mistake.

While many nursing homes may look like hospitals, may seem to function like hospitals, may even smell like hospitals, they are not hospitals. They are primarily places of residence for a unique population of people who need a place to live that also provides care. You are visiting your relative in his or her place of residence, and you will need to conduct your visits accordingly.

Stop a minute and consider what would go on when you saw Mom at her apartment or home. Did you walk into the home and hug her? Did you feel compelled to talk nonstop from the minute you entered the room? Did you do things together in the house? out of the house? Did you go for lunch or take her to have her hair done? When there was a lull in the conversation, did it feel natural?

Now think about your visits to Mom at the nursing home. How are you feeling before you get there? guilty? upset? Do the visits drag along because the two of you have run out of things to say? Are you seeing her more often then you ever did when she lived at home?

Successful visiting takes planning. Suggestions gathered from nursing home staff, other caregivers, and residents themselves may help you in formulating a style that will make your visits therapeutic not only for your relative but for you as well.

1. Visit during meals. This can serve a number of purposes. If your relative is disoriented and needs help with feeding, this is a loving, caring act you can perform. If your relative is alert and capable, he or she will love showing you off to other residents and staff.
2. Attend some regularly scheduled event at the nursing home together. If your relative can no longer get out for religious services, attend services at the home with him or her.
3. Get out of the room. Ask the person to give you a tour of the home if that is feasible; suggest a treat at the snack shop; take the person "shopping" at the resident store— "I need a gift for Martha's birthday next week."
4. If possible, get out of the building. Go out to eat, go to a mall at a quiet time of the day or evening. Attend a community event. Go for a drive. And when you go out to eat, go to the same restaurant at the same time of day so that the restaurant staff begins to recognize you and your relative.
5. If you or someone else in the family has talent, volunteer to do a program for the residents. On your relative's actual birthday, make a big deal of the event. (Most homes have monthly birthday parties in which all residents with birthdays that month are honored on the same day.)
6. When you sit quietly and talk, focus on those topics that were natural in the past. If your relative loved gossip,

share the local gossip. If you depended on Dad for financial advice, seek his advice now. Talk about children and grandchildren who are away at school or living in other communities. Bring in snapshots.

7. Do something with/for the resident. Occasionally help him or her change the decor of the room. Read the newspaper aloud. Clean out the closet and dresser and change clothes from winter to summer just as you used to at home. Give your Mom a manicure. One caregiver told how once a week she would come with her kit for doing a manicure and spend an hour working with her mother's nails. In this time there was little need for detailed conversation. They just enjoyed a quiet time together.

8. Show by your attention that you take this person seriously even when his or her impairment makes understanding difficult.

9. If illness leaves the person unable to carry on conversation, comfort by giving the person a massage or brushing his or her hair.

10. Do not use visits as occasions to give advice or scold the resident or to downgrade the staff. If your relative has a complaint, listen and assure him or her that you will follow through.

Finally, let your relative see that you are maintaining an active association with the home and thereby with your relative. If the home has a support group, attend the meetings. If there is a family council, become involved. If neither group exists, explore organizing them for your relative's home.

And if you live in another town and can only visit on rare occasions, maintain contact with lots of short notes, cards, snapshots, news clippings, letters from your children, and phone calls.

What about holidays and other special events? If possible, include the person in the day's events in the traditional way. Take him or her to your home for the day or out to dinner if that is the tradition, or bring the holiday to your relative. Include your relative in the preparations for the holiday. Work on cards together. If it is an occasion such as a wedding or graduation in the family, bring some of the planning work with you when you visit and enlist the help of your relative. If it is an occasion for gifts, work together on the resident's gift list and shopping. If he or she cannot go out to choose gifts, bring a selection in and let the person choose. Do the wrapping *with* your relative, not for him or her (even if all the person can do is observe and make an occasional comment).

Gifts for the Nursing Home Resident

Speaking of gifts, what on earth can you give someone who is living in a limited space and who already has had to cut back considerably on personal possessions? There are more ideas than you might expect for appropriate gifts for nursing home residents.

Start with utilitarian needs. Does the person use a walker or wheelchair? Does he or she have a carryall bag that fits on the device allowing him or her to carry along glasses, tissues, a changepurse, even a paperback book or extra sweater? Or, if the person spends a great deal of time in bed, consider a bedside caddy. This is a colorful fabric strip with pockets to hold items the person might want handy. One end of the strip fits between the mattress and springs, and the part with the pocket hangs on the side within easy reach.

There are other practical gifts as well. You may wish to write for the following catalogs, which specialize in articles for the disabled:

- Fred Sammons Inc., Box 32, Brookfield IL 60513 (1-800-323-7305)
- Cleo Living Aids, 3058 Mayfield Rd., Cleveland OH 44121 (1-800-321-0595)
- Comfortably Yours, 61 West Hunter Avenue, Maywood, NJ 07607.

For those who ask, you might suggest the following gifts: stamped envelopes, a selection of cards, an up-to-date address book, subscriptions, library books (also large-print books or magazine editions), toilet items, clothing, costume jewelry for the ladies, a small window bird feeder (has suction cups to attach it to the resident's window) and some birdseed in a covered container, writing supplies, a lap desk, a tape recording of a family gathering, scrapbooks, stained glass window ornaments, a night light, "talking" books (books read aloud on tape), Walkman® tape player and/or radio with earphones (also earphones for television).

And what do you avoid? Foods, especially things that are not on the person's diet. Anything that takes up space—space in the person's room is limited. Clothing that is impractical or needs special care. Expensive or valuable jewelry or keepsakes that could disappear (even if they do not disappear, they can be a constant source of worry and anxiety for the person). Plants may seem perfect but are often a nuisance, requiring care the resident cannot give and the staff has little time for.

And what do residents themselves suggest? One survey of nursing home residents indicated that they considered the very best gifts to be:

- visits
- phone calls
- greeting cards with handwritten messages
- anything created by a grandchild
- outings
- warm-up suits
- socks
- housecoats
- anything that makes them laugh

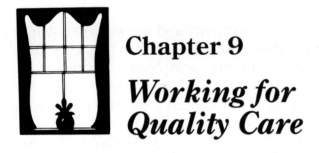

Chapter 9

Working for Quality Care

In any situation where numbers of people live together, problems are going to arise. In a situation where those people are impaired and in need of a high level of care, problems are inevitable.

You can expect that you and your relative are not always going to be thrilled with life in the nursing home. Sometimes there are going to be problems, complaints, and causes for concern. In the best homes, such issues will be met honestly and rectified immediately. Your role as a caregiver includes the responsibility of monitoring care, and in this role you are responsible for presenting any concerns to the appropriate parties for consideration. Keep in mind that you are monitoring one individual, while the staff is responsible for many. You also need to keep in mind that some problems have no solutions. A nursing home cannot make a dying person well.

In order to successfully monitor care, keep in mind the following checklist:

• Take seriously any complaint presented by your relative, but do not assume the worst. Oversights and mistakes are going to happen. The care the person received at home was not perfect; it will not be perfect in a nursing home.

• Read the section on handling complaints and problems on pages 134–140 and follow the suggested procedures in voicing your concerns.

• Visit often and at various times of the day and night.

• If your relative has a complaint that you can check out yourself, do so. (See page 136.)

• Check with staff before you become alarmed by any complaint your relative makes. This shows that you are interested in giving staff an opportunity to explain the situation, that you are interested in working with them, that you understand there are two sides to every story.

• Take note of not only your relative but his or her roommate and other residents as well. Because you are there and the staff knows your relative has someone who cares, they may give better care. Observe those residents who have no one and see how the staff cares for them.

• Take note of personal grooming care: Is your relative clean, are nails clean and clipped, is mouth fresh (teeth brushed), is hair combed, is the person appropriately dressed? Accompany your relative to the bathroom or offer to give a backrub and check for skin breakdown that could lead to bedsores.

• If there is a change in your relative's mental health that the staff automatically attributes to dementia, be concerned. Many causes of mental impairment in older persons are treatable.

• If you do not receive satisfaction by working through the staff at the home, contact the ombudsperson.

A person who moves into a nursing home becomes a resident in a new place with new neighbors and new people providing services. It will take time to adjust—from all sides. The staff will need to adjust to your relative at the same time he or she and you are adjusting to them.

How Can You Work with the Staff?

Face it, you will have some doubts and suspicions about the quality of care your relative is going to receive in this home. Even though you have made what you think is the best possible choice, it may still be the better of two or more evils in your eyes. If your attitude toward nursing homes is basically one of mistrust and antipathy, you may enter this relationship with staff on a less than positive note. So, the chief question is how to get the best care possible for your relative. Do you present yourself to the staff as the squeaky wheel or the sweetheart? Do you nag or do you cajole?

You should not have to be or do either. You should be able to build a relationship with staff personnel based on your mutual interest in providing the best possible care for your relative. Of course, you will need to understand that your mission is to get that care for one person—your relative—while theirs is to provide that care for as many residents as are admitted to the facility.

Author Doug Manning says, "It is amazing how much more we criticize when we are spectators instead of participants. It is also amazing how much more effective criticism can be when it comes from a participant."[1]

Begin with the positives: The members of the staff at the facility you have chosen are first and foremost human beings. Many of them have elderly parents of their own. Many of them got into this field of work because they genuinely like people. Many of them—from the administrator to the nursing assistant—believe they can make a difference.

In a long-term care setting, staff members are far more intimately involved with residents (and their families) than they would be if they worked in a hospital. These people are going to get to know your relative and your relative is going to get to know them on a personal level. As you visit over weeks and months, certain staff members will become familiar to you. You will call them by name and know details of their lives as they will know details of yours. In a manner of speaking, you and the staff will become colleagues in providing a plan of care for your relative.

To compare this situation to the hospital setting in another way, in the hospital setting family members are often largely ignored, even rebuffed when they try to participate

---

[1]D. Manning, *When Love Gets Tough: The Nursing Home Decision* (Hereford, TX: In-Sight Books, 1983).

in the care of a relative. In the nursing home, they can become welcome members of the care team.

The Team

As you have learned, the nursing staff (assistants, staff nurses, charge nurse, director of nursing) and therapists carry out a medical plan prescribed by the physician. Because they work closely with the resident, these are the people who have the best opportunity to notice changes in his or her condition and needs. The nursing staff along with the social worker are also responsible for relaying information to family and for letting family caregivers know when the resident has needs the family can meet.

The social services staff—activity personnel, social workers, and others—are responsible for coordinating a program of care that meets the needs of each resident for mental stimulation and worthwhile activity throughout the day.

The administrator is responsible for overseeing the entire operation of the home, including services provided by in-house staff and those provided by outside agencies or persons. He or she sets the tone for the home and is usually the key to the quality of care and programming the home will offer a resident.

And you are responsible for acting as a liaison between your relative and the staff when necessary, for providing information that can help the staff in providing the best care for your relative, and for overseeing the quality of that care and its administration.

If more than one family member is involved, decide who will speak for the family. Make certain the family is in agreement before you try to address concerns you may have about your relative's care. A family in conflict only makes life more difficult for everyone—including the resident.

The Ground Rules

A few basics may help you in getting off on the right foot:

1. Understand what roles individual staff persons play within the home. While hopefully you will never encounter an

attitude of "That's not my job," it will help if you can understand the difference between a charge nurse and a director of nursing, for example, and know who to approach in what circumstance.

2. The stated goal of any long-term facility is to assist residents in achieving as much independence as possible within the confines of their impairments. You may encounter instances where you think your relative is not getting enough help. Do not assume someone is not doing his or her job. Instead, ask about the plan for your relative. Perhaps your mother is not being assisted in buttoning her blouse because the physical therapist said the action would be good exercise for her fingers. The point is not to assume poor care until you have investigated.

3. If you expect courtesy and respect for your relative, you will need to deliver courtesy and respect to those who provide care for him or her. And if necessary, you will need to see that your relative also gives the staff courtesy and respect. These people are trained professionals, even those who provide the most basic care; they are not servants.

4. If you want the right to criticize, you will need to offer praise when it is due.

5. If you want the staff to listen to you, you will have to give them the courtesy of listening to their ideas as well.

6. Members of the staff are not mindreaders. They will get to know your relative sooner and better if you take the time to give them information that may help in their care plan. At the same time, showing your interest in getting to know individual staff persons as individuals will get your relative better care every time.

7. If your relative was difficult or abusive at home, he or she is likely to be difficult or abusive in the nursing home. Your understanding and support for the staff can go a long way toward their providing better care for your relative.

Your relative is not going to receive the high level of one-to-one care he or she received at home. As a caregiver, you know how demanding the role is. You know that when you try to describe it, the job sounds fairly simple and even minor. And yet, you have experienced firsthand how time-consuming and demanding caring for an older person with multiple frailties can be. Multiply your experience by three or four or ten and you begin to understand the role of giving care as a long-term care facility staff person. Attention needs to be given to all residents who need assistance in moving from bed to chair, in walking, in getting to and from the bathroom. Not one but many residents are incontinent and must be changed not once but several times throughout a day. And on top of being needed to meet these basic requirements for daily physical and personal care, staff members must also be prepared to care for the many mentally confused residents who insist on leaving, who cling, who cry out, and who need constant reassurance.

There is no question that there has been a history of poor care in many nursing homes in the United States. But there are good homes with dedicated employees, and even in the best of homes staff members may sometimes experience what has been called "emotional atrophy."

No wonder they perform better when there is some recognition and understanding from families of the vital work they do. You, of all people, can understand that. You have been and are a caregiver. You must remember times when someone's unexpected expression of respect and praise boosted your morale and gave you the motivation to press on with the hard task of giving care.

How Do You Assess the Home's Performance?

One of the reactions you are going to have in these first weeks is wondering whether you made the right choice. You had only a couple of homes to choose from, and the time for evaluating them was so short and pressured. Is this the best choice?

The first question to ask yourself is whether those terms that are placed in the admissions contract are being fulfilled. If therapy was prescribed, is it being delivered? on time? as many times as originally prescribed? What services were included in that basic care cost? Is every service being delivered?

By the way, you have some responsibility here, too. If the home calls and says they are meeting about your relative on Tuesday, make it your business to be there on Tuesday if at all possible. Also, if the home has regularly scheduled sessions where family members have an opportunity to meet with staff members and discuss concerns, attend at least some of those sessions. You do not always have to go in with a complaint or concern. It would be lovely if at least one time you showed up simply to say what a good job the staff was doing.

There are a few indicators that will give you some reassurance immediately:

- Did the home's staff make a care plan for your relative?
- Was your relative a party to the formulation of that plan? were you?
- Does the home make provision for regular meetings with the family member to go over the resident's progress and care plan and make any adjustments and hear any concerns?
- Does the staff encourage your involvement with the care of your relative?
- Does the staff listen when you ask questions and receive your concerns as genuine rather than nuisances?
- Does the home's staff seem to work hard to foster independence on whatever level is possible, or do you see signs that they are really too helpful to residents?
- Do they infantilize residents with pet names and lack of basic respect such as knocking before entering the resident's room? (You should have noticed this in your initial tour.)
- Do you see teaching going on with the staff?
- Are there signs that this home seeks innovative ways of making life better for all residents through the use of novel and creative programming?

An example of innovative programming is the home that asked residents who were relatively independent and capable to act as a welcoming committee for new residents on a rotating basis. A member of the committee would greet the new resident and his or her family, show them the ropes, make certain the new resident had a place in the dining room and met other residents, etc. The plan is simple but enormously effective in that it places the new resident in a position of dealing with his or her peers immediately without the intervention of staff and in that the entrenched resident gets a chance to show off his or her knowledge and pride in the home.

You also have time now to evaluate some of the extra services you may not have had time to look at before. These services may include eye care, where glasses are regularly cleaned and checked for proper fit, and the same attention to dentures and hearing aids. You also will want to take a close look at basic hygiene: foot care especially if your relative is diabetic; manicures especially if the person has had a stroke and has a contracted hand; hair care—even without using the beauty/barber shop, hair can be clean and combed; and skin care—old skin is fragile and should be treated that way, tenderly and with care beyond simple washing and drying.

Another indicator of good care is when a home places some value on counseling services for both the resident and the family. Is mental health considered an important piece of the healthcare puzzle at the home? even for those who have been diagnosed as having some dementia? Even dementia patients can feel depression and anger. And while it is difficult to counsel someone who has memory defects, it is possible to show some understanding of his or her mental pain in the same way you would acknowledge physical pain in someone else.

Do family members take advantage of opportunities to meet together in a support group? Are families clearly an integral part of the nursing home's team? After a time, assuming you are visiting regularly, you should expect at least some staff persons to address you by name and to recognize you beyond being Mr. Smith's daughter.

Speaking of visiting, keep your eyes open when you do. What goes on and, if it is upsetting to you, does it happen regularly or were you just there on a bad day? For example, even staff persons regularly complain about the physician who makes his visits to the residents by simply sticking his head in the door (without knocking) and asking "How are we doing today?" before moving on to the next room. And this is a *staff* complaint. Residents are supposed to be assessed by the physician on a regular basis. You have the right to expect that this assessment will go beyond waving in the door and glancing at a chart at the nurses' station.

This example should show you that while there is no question staff can be inattentive and even indifferent to the individual needs of each resident, there are individual staff members in many homes who share your concerns. They get upset when your father's favorite sweater gets lost in the laundry, just as you do. They are stunned by the amount of time they are expected to give to filling out forms and recording information when they could be giving care to residents. They may agree that your aunt is oversedated and be as concerned as you are that something be done.

In short, if you learn to work with the staff and the home instead of assuming the worst, you could make life better for everyone. As a part of a team effort, you might even be able to improve the system.

But What about Poor Care?

Poor care results when needs for assistance, protection, security, and mental, emotional, and physical well-being are neglected and unmet.

Abuse—subtle, overt, intended, and accidental—happens. And it happens for all sorts of reasons. Sometimes the reasons are within your control. Most of the time they are not. Sometimes poor care comes from administrative problems. Understaffing for any reason can lead even dedicated people to make mistakes, deliver less than good care, or take measures that are designed for the convenience of the staff rather than the well-being of the resident (use of restraints is an example).

Inadequate training is another problem. A nursing assistant who is thrown in to sink or swim with minimal or no preparation for handling frail older persons is a disaster waiting to happen. Staff persons who receive little incentive, continuing education, and/or praise for the work they do can develop attitude and morale problems that lead to poor care.

Physical abuse is the one that usually makes the headlines, but there are all sorts of manifestations of poor delivery of long-term care. Certainly abrasions, lacerations, fractures, bruises, burns, and any other physical evidence of poor care need to be investigated. But you also need to be aware of the more subtle evidence. If your relative shows signs of depression, a sudden onset of inappropriate behavior, or poor hygiene, or if you observe excessive use of medication for purposes of sedation or restraint, untreated medical problems, or failure to respond to concerns (yours or the resident's), you must consider the possibility of abuse.

One of the most common—and damaging—forms of abuse in long-term care is simple neglect of the most basic care. Medical attention may be given, but meeting the person's needs in the areas of hygiene, nutrition, fluid intake, and opportunities for activity are postponed because the staff is overworked, too busy, or simply unconcerned.

The four most frequently reported problems of abuse in nursing homes are infantilization, depersonalization, dehumanization, and victimization.[2] In addition to those issues, you will need to concern yourself with discrimination that can occur particularly when the resident's pay source is Title XIX (Medicaid). If you suspect your relative is being discriminated against on the basis of payment source, you may wish to write for the report, "Medicaid Discrimination in Long Term Care," available from the National Citizens' Coalition for Nursing Home Reform (1424 Sixteenth Street NW, Suite L-2, Washington, DC 20036-2211).

---

[2]A. Monk, L. W. Kaye, and H. Litwin, *Resolving Grievances in the Nursing Home: A Study of the Ombudsman Program* (New York: Columbia University Press, 1984), p. 4.

How Do You Handle Complaints?

If you have not done so already, take a good look at the written statement of your relative's rights as a resident of the nursing home. Basic rights mandated federally are listed in Appendix B on page 161.

Any institution, as you have seen, must function within the parameters of a set of guidelines that are created to provide the best care and services for the most residents. Therefore, the traditional nursing home setting may seem particularly confining especially in those first weeks of residency. For someone who is used to getting something from the kitchen or going for a walk whenever he or she wishes, these rules can seem unfair. As a family member, you will need to listen carefully to your relative's complaints and to keep your eyes and ears open when you visit. You understand that there must be some limitations. However, limiting a person's freedom simply because it is inconvenient for the staff to honor that freedom is not acceptable and should not be tolerated.

Residents themselves have spoken out about quality of care in a report published by the National Citizens' Coalition for Nursing Home Reform. Some of their conclusions were:

- "choices and the right to make them are primary markers of quality care"
- "a pleasing and happy homelike atmosphere is desirable"
- "good feelings and attitudes between residents and all levels of staff, and among residents, are essential to quality care."
- "individualization and personalization rank high . . . residents say they want as much independence as possible, whatever their level of ability and they want the opportunity to help themselves whenever possible"
- "for the less able [residents] identify the need for more care, visitors and attention"[3]

---

[3]From NCCNHR Summary Report, April 1985, "A Consumer Perspective on Quality Care: The Residents' Point of View," p. 14.

Most commonly the complaint will be about something small: "The aide doesn't come when I ring." "The food is lousy." "I don't like my roommate." "They lost my favorite nightgown in the laundry."

It may help you to know what residents see as their primary needs for a good life in a nursing home. Clifford Bennett[4] lists the priority of needs by importance as:

- possessions
- family
- freedom
- privacy
- independence
- making decisions
- choice of food
- friends
- choice of what to wear
- religion
- control over own financial affairs
- communication with people outside the home
- recognition
- community activities
- shopping and buying
- accomplishment

And yet the likelihood of your relative voicing his or her own complaint is slim. Residents do not complain for any number of reasons: "I don't want to be a bother." "I'm afraid they won't like me." "It's a little thing—I can live with it." "I'm afraid they might do something to me."

Retaliation in any form—overt or subtle—is against the law, but do not be naive. It happens. You complain about the bruise on your mother's arm to the charge nurse. She reprimands the assistant. The assistant gets upset and when your mother rings her call bell for help in getting to the bathroom, the assistant does not hurry to answer the bell.

---

[4]C. Bennett, *Nursing Home Life: What It Is and What It Could Be* (New York: The Tiresias Press, Inc. 1980), p. 37.

Your mother soils herself. The assistant reprimands your mother for making a mess. That is retaliation.

Or you have a number of concerns about your wife's care that you take to the administrator. You see that he has labeled you as a troublemaker, and, while he promises to see that these matters are addressed, nothing happens. You take your complaints to the ombudsperson who follows through and assists you in getting matters straightened out for your wife. Then your wife goes to the hospital for a few weeks. When she returns to the home, the administrator informs her that it was necessary to move her to another floor and room. This is retaliation.

So what can you do to ensure good care and to make things better when good care is not present?

Talk First

"I know you are busy but when you have a minute could we talk about . . . ?" Or, "I'd really be grateful if . . . ." The idea is to ask rather than demand, to talk about a concern rather than assume a problem. Since most of your relative's care is being given by nursing assistants, try to get to know them as individuals and to enlist them in your plan to get the best possible care for your relative. "What do you think?" can work miracles sometimes.

Follow the Hierarchy

When your best efforts at treating all staff as colleagues fail, start going up the ladder. Take the problem to the most logical source. If your mother cannot drink milk and yet milk consistently appears with her meal, go to the dietician or person in charge of food service. Always take the approach that this is a mistake that is happening this once. You are certain it will be cleared up. "I know you have so many individual diets, but if milk comes with her meal, Mom is going to drink it and that is going to be a medical problem. Can you make sure it doesn't happen again?"

Another example: Your father's good flannel shirts keep disappearing in the laundry. Go to the head of housekeeping. "I have a problem. Dad's shirts never seem to come back from the laundry. I'm spending a fortune replacing them. Is there a problem with the way I'm marking them or is there something else I can do to make certain he gets them back?" You are not accusing anyone of anything. You are asking for some advice and help.

If you get no results with this sort of positive attitude, move up the ladder all the way to the administrator if necessary or to the director of nursing (if the matter involves medical care).

Take Advantage of Opportunities to Interact with Staff

As you have learned, in many homes family members are invited to attend regular staffing sessions. At these meetings, family members are encouraged to participate in reevaluation of the care plan for their relative and to express any concerns they may have. A caregiver who shows his or her concern and interest by attending these sessions whenever possible is a caregiver who is likely to get results. You may find out that one or more of the staff shares your concern and is interested in taking steps to make matters better.

There will be other opportunities for interacting with staff, and you should take advantage of any you can. Many homes sponsor open houses periodically throughout the year as well as parties and banquets for special occasions.

Talk to Other Family Members and Residents

If several of you are having the same problem, you'll find strength in numbers. Also, you may discover that the director of nursing, administrator, or other senior staff will actually appreciate your bringing a problem to his or her attention. These people may be dedicated, but they cannot be everywhere at once.

If you have reason to believe that a particular problem affects several residents in the home, you may wish to speak with other family members. Concerted action from a group may sometimes bring better and quicker results than the voice of one person. As an individual or a group, be certain you know what it is you want before you send your representative to complain. Consider the following questions as guidelines:

- What is the problem?
- What would make it better?
- What specific action do you want taken?
- What if that is impossible? Do you have an alternative idea?

Know Your Relative's Resident Rights

These are not just high-minded statements put together by dedicated and concerned professionals. These are guarantees by law.

Consider the matter of transfers. There are only four reasons the institution may instigate proceedings for transfer or discharge: for the resident's own welfare, for the safety of others, for nonpayment, or in the case where the resident was admitted as a Medicare patient and is no longer in need of skilled care Medicare covers (in this case the resident will transfer to a bed in another unit of the home). On the subject of nonpayment, your relative may not be discharged or transferred for nonpayment simply because his or her private funds have run out and he or she is now entitled to Medicaid (unless the home is not certified to receive Medicaid).

And yet transfers take place all the time that are suspiciously tied to just such a circumstance as change in source of payment. "They are not supposed to transfer but they do," one hospital social worker stated. "Some places are really good at finding a reason for admitting the person to the hospital just about the time money is running out. The majority bend over backwards to take their own back, but occasionally you can see it all coming together—the hospitalization just at the exact time the private funds are running out and then the declaration that there are no Title XIX beds available."

When All Else Fails, Call the
Office of the State Ombudsperson

The ombudsperson program was established for just this purpose—to assist residents and family members in overseeing the care provided by long-term care facilities. By law, the ombudsperson is required to follow up on all complaints without revealing the source of the complaint unless given permission to do so.

As you have seen, your attitude will be very important in how your complaints will be received. Sometimes a caregiver who feels enormous guilt will work through that guilt by finding fault with everything the staff does. This person may be looking for someone else to blame for the fact that his or her relative has had to come to this facility. All caregivers need to understand that there are going to be problems and there are going to be two sides to every story.

Example: One caregiver was hysterical when she arrived late one Sunday morning to find her mother still in her night clothes lying in bed. Without stopping to speak to her mother, she charged up to the nurses' station where several staff members were gathered and demanded to know why they were loafing around.

An assistant accompanied her to her mother's room where the older woman greeted her daughter with a delighted smile and said, "Isn't this grand, dear? Sunday morning—breakfast in bed and the *New York Times!* Just like home."

When a problem does arise, be aware of your tone and approach. This is not the time to put people on the defensive. No one responds well to accusations. If possible, take notes of the conversation, then if something that is promised is not forthcoming you have the notes to back you up. By all means, go out of your way to solve the problem in-house before approaching outside mediators. If you run to the state ombudsperson with every little grievance, the home's staff is not going to be terribly responsive to your relative's needs.

When you have a problem, begin by asking why it happens the way it does, what options for change are available, and what it would take to have things done the way you want them.

You will probably hear excuses such as: "We were short-staffed that day." Or, "It's hard to take care of that in the morning when we're so swamped." Or, "We can't do that— the state won't let us."

Maybe. But if you hear the same excuse again and again, it is time to consider at least speaking with the ombudsperson and seeing what your next step needs to be. According to the study conducted by the Institute of Medicine prior to the passage of the reform act of 1987, "Ombudsmen help individual residents and their families negotiate with nursing homes and regulatory agencies."[5] The ombudsperson is there to work with individuals, and his or her focus is on solving problems rather than on finding fault and placing blame. Think of this office as consumer representatives.

For the most part, people who work in long-term care are good people, trying hard to do a good job under sometimes adverse conditions. Be reasonable in your expectations. If your relative's behavior can be a problem (and you know this because you lived with it yourself during all those months and years of caregiving), do not expect miracles.

In her sociological look at life in nursing homes, Joan Retsinas notes, "the family that pointedly commiserates with staff, that shows some compassion toward them and that occasionally expresses gratitude may help distraught staff better serve an otherwise difficult patient. Indeed, staff may grow fond of Mom, and when she leaves, they will miss her."[6]

[5]Institute of Medicine, Committee on Nursing Home Regulation, *Improving the Quality of Care in Nursing Homes* (Washington, DC: National Academy Press, 1986), p. 178.

[6]J. Retsinas, *It's Okay, Mom: The Nursing Home from a Sociological Perspective* (New York: The Tiresias Press, Inc., 1986).

Chapter 10

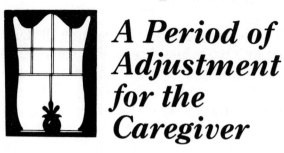

A Period of Adjustment for the Caregiver

You are still a caregiver even though the person has moved to another level of care. You are still needed and your role is still vital. Now that the dust has settled a bit, it is time to consider one other person in this matter. You. Your concentration has been on your relative and the performance of the staff at the home you have chosen. You may have spent some time trying to help other family members adjust to the idea that a loved one now resides in a nursing home. You have been busy trying to get everything set to make this as positive an experience as possible.

As a caregiver, you are going to go through your own period of adjustment. You will need and deserve support and help during this difficult time. Especially if the person now living in a nursing home is your spouse, you need to seek some help in making the transition that comes when people who have been married for many years find themselves living apart.

How Do You Feel?

One caregiver reminisced about those first days when she finally had time to understand that not only had her father's life changed but her own had as well. "It's a relief and then immediately, there is guilt. You think, 'How can I feel that way—relieved?'"

And there are other feelings—loneliness, especially if the relative now living in the nursing home is a spouse. "Our social network did not stay in place once he became ill. Our friends were uncomfortable with his illness. For some time I was too occupied with taking care of him to notice how everyone had drifted away, but now . . . ."

In some cases there is anger. "Our son does not go to visit unless I practically beg him. He says, 'My father has been gone for some time now. Why should I go?'" Or, "My mother is always pleasant to the staff but she barely speaks to me. When I went there on Christmas she told every staff person, 'Merry Christmas,' as I walked with her through the halls, but she never once said it to me."

And the new American family structure cannot be underestimated as a contributing factor to this issue. In today's society, divorce and remarriage are common. This can blur the lines of responsibility especially in cases where the daughter-in-law was the primary caregiver. There is also the factor of distance and mobility. Families are spread out over greater distances. On-site caregiving sometimes is simply not possible.

How Can You Cope?

The first coping mechanism is understanding that you are still a caregiver, you are still needed. Your role has not ended; it has simply changed. Caregivers and professionals offer the following coping techniques:

1. Understand that it is possible the decision was never even in your hands to begin with. The person's physician or other family members or complicated circumstances may have demanded a higher level of care than you could possibly have provided. What you have done in finding a nursing home for your relative may well have been an act of love and caring.
2. Continue to give care. There are both meaningful and meaningless ways to do this. Meaningless ways include keeping a vigil at the nursing home as if by being there practically all the time you may be able to prevent some

tragedy or alleviate your guilt. Another meaningless involvement is overprotecting your relative—doing everything for him or her instead of allowing the home to foster whatever independence is possible.

Meaningful ways include finding activities that keep you involved in the person's new life while at the same time allowing the person to accept his or her new circumstances. These activities include doing the person's personal laundry so that there is a familiar touch and smell of home; performing small personal care tasks such as shining shoes, combing hair, washing dentures and/or eyeglasses when you visit; taking the person out or accompanying him or her to events in the nursing home.

3. Ask the staff what you might do to help your relative when you visit. Learn to assist with the physical therapy exercises; encourage your relative to attend programs; come at mealtime and help with feeding if that is a part of care.

4. Give of yourself to the community within the home. Volunteer. Present a program. Bring in programs from the community. Enlist the support and participation of those clubs and organizations to which you belong.

5. Organize a family council (if there isn't already one) to complement the home's resident council. Family councils provide a means to bring problems and concerns to the attention of the administration, to assist in planning programming for the residents, to make suggestions for improvements in management and programming, to offer support and counseling for family members, to advocate outside the home for better conditions and standards and for financial supports.

6. If you have been the primary caregiver for a person who is now residing in a nursing home, it is time to take charge of your life. Your relative has a whole new routine to get used to. The nursing home offers potential friendships, new hobbies, an enjoyable social life, and rehabilitation. He or she does not need you for everything as in the past. You need to think about what will fill your life now. "I went to work," one caregiver announced. "I need to be

needed after all these years of caring for Papa. I haven't worked in 35 years but it gets me out and I'm with people and I do forget."

7. Get involved on a large scale. Become a spokesperson for this growing population that cannot speak for itself. Help organize a community nursing home council.

How Can You Make a Difference?

"Ultimately the prevention of inadequate care of the elderly is a political issue," say Terry T. Fulmer and Terrence A. O'Malley.[1] "Abuse and neglect will diminish when society places a higher value on the well-being of its elderly citizens."

There are a number of ways in which others work to protect the rights of nursing home residents. In addition to the ombudsperson program, resident councils, and family councils, consumer advocacy groups and volunteer advocates have been very instrumental in making life better for those in need of institutional long-term care.

The time is ripe for change. The passage of the nursing home reforms of 1987 was a major milestone in advocacy for these people. Americans are beginning to wake up to the fact that the older population is growing faster than any other segment of the population. For the first time in the history of the nation, there are more people over the age of 65 than there are teenagers.

So, the answer to the question, "What can one caregiver do?" is moot. You are not one caregiver against the world. There are literally hundreds of thousands of you out there. Many of you as members of the largest segment of the population—the Baby Boomers—already have real power. You vote in extraordinary numbers, you are better educated than any generation that has preceded you, and you have learned how to use the system so that it works for you.

And as experienced caregivers, you have expertise that many of those making policy do not have.

[1]T. T. Fulmer and T. A. O'Malley, *Inadequate Care of the Elderly: A Health Care Perspective on Abuse and Neglect* (New York: Springer Publishing Co., 1987), p. 152.

What Needs Doing?

"Where to begin?" may be a better question. In a 1983 report, the National Citizens' Coalition for Nursing Home Reform found that:

- The median age for nursing home residents was 81 years.
- Residents have an average of four medical conditions affecting their health.
- An estimated 32 percent are impaired by mental confusion.
- More than half the residents have no regular visitors.
- Almost half of the residents are childless.
- Over 70 percent are female.[2]

Clearly this is a vulnerable population, mostly incapable of speaking out for themselves. Add to that the fact that everyone is aging and you may see the importance of working now for systems and programs that will ensure a higher quality of care and lifestyle in the future.

In the report that led to the sweeping reforms enacted by Congress in December 1987, the Institute of Medicine stated that, "Three . . . sets of factors affect quality of care and quality of life in nursing homes: (1) consumer involvement and consumer advocacy, (2) community interest and involvement in nursing homes, and (3) the motivation, attitudes and qualifications of nursing home management and staff . . . . Active participation by the residents in some aspects of management policy and care decisions can have important effects on quality of care and quality of life."[3]

A 1987 survey conducted by the American Association of Retired Persons and the Villers Foundation found that one in two Americans will spend some time in a nursing home

---

[2]National Citizens' Coalition for Nursing Home Reform, *Consumer Statement of Principles for the Nursing Home Regulatory System—State Licensure and Federal Certification Programs* (Washington, DC: NCCNHR, September 1983), p. 53.

[3]Institute of Medicine, *Improving the Quality of Care in Nursing Homes* (National Academy Press: Washington, DC, 1986), p. 19.

at one point in their lives. The absence of a national long-term care policy is seen by U.S. families as a national crisis. Sixty percent of the one thousand people surveyed reported some personal experience with the need for long-term care. Four in ten experienced difficulty in paying for that care. And a 1988 report of the House Select Committee on Aging indicates that half of the couples with one spouse in a nursing home become impoverished within six months and 70 percent of single elderly patients reach the poverty level after 13 weeks in a nursing home.

Many nursing homes throughout the country are consistently understaffed, and the staff that is present is undertrained. Because reimbursement rates are low, pay scales for staff in nursing homes is correspondingly low, and there is little money available for programming that could motivate staff to better care. (One state pays $100 per day for prisoners and $60 a day for Title XIX care in a nursing home.)

And the list goes on.

What Are the Suggested Solutions?

The National Citizens Coalition for Nursing Home Reform (NCCNHR) suggests that the best homes operate under a "resident-focused" system. (See Figure 10-1.)

For the overall quality of nursing home care as an important piece of the total long-term care picture, a community-based approach is advocated. The nursing home industry alone should not be expected to provide all the services necessary to assure quality of life for its residents any more than any one segment or industry in the community would be expected to fulfill all the needs of the citizens living there.

Figure 10-1 How a resident-focused system should function

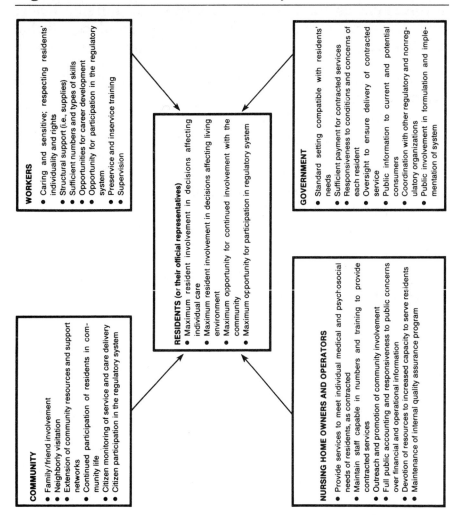

WORKERS

- Caring and sensitive; respecting residents' individuality and rights
- Structural support (i.e., supplies)
- Sufficient numbers and types of skills
- Opportunities for career development
- Opportunity for participation in the regulatory system
- Preservice and inservice training
- Supervision

GOVERNMENT

- Standard setting compatible with residents' needs
- Sufficient payment for contracted services
- Responsiveness to conditions and concerns of each resident
- Oversight to ensure delivery of contracted service
- Public information to current and potential consumers
- Coordination with other regulatory and nonregulatory organizations
- Public involvement in formulation and implementation of system

RESIDENTS (or their official representatives)

- Maximum resident involvement in decisions affecting individual care
- Maximum resident involvement in decisions affecting living environment
- Maximum opportunity for continued involvement with the community
- Maximum opportunity for participation in regulatory system

COMMUNITY

- Family/friend involvement
- Neighborly visitation
- Extension of community resources and support networks
- Continued participation of residents in community life
- Citizen monitoring of service and care delivery
- Citizen participation in the regulatory system

NURSING HOME OWNERS AND OPERATORS

- Provide services to meet individual medical and psychosocial needs of residents, as contracted
- Maintain staff capable in numbers and training to provide contracted services
- Outreach and promotion of community involvement
- Full public accounting and responsiveness to public concerns over financial and operational information
- Devotion of resources to increased capacity to serve residents
- Maintenance of internal quality assurance program

SOURCE: National Citizens' Coalition for Nursing Home Reform, 1983.

AARP's volunteer organization targets community involvement as the key to quality of life in nursing homes and other long-term care facilities. The group advocates that the following objectives be addressed by community leaders:[4]

• educate citizens in and out of nursing homes about residents' rights
• facilitate new inspection procedure
• set up a community nursing home council to work with nursing home staff and residents to improve conditions
• foster intergenerational activities that bring younger people into the nursing home, educating them about the importance of long-term care
• encourage recognition of residents, staff, and volunteers throughout the community

The NCCNHR suggests the following possibilities for community involvement in better care and quality of life for long-term care facility residents:[5]

TOTAL COMMUNITY APPROACH
Selected Example Activities

Religious Institutions, Organizations and Related Groups
• Churches, synagogues, clubs can "adopt a nursing home," for visitation, other special services (such as religious ceremonies, provision of clothing, transportation to church and to other community functions); personal religious counseling or emotional support services; utilization of nursing home residents as volunteers for the church, etc.

Libraries
• Reading and audio-visual services and programs for residents in the facility

---

[4]American Association of Retired Persons, "Community Involvement Increases the Quality of Life in Local Nursing Homes," *Highlights*, Vol. 6, No. 2 (May 1988), p. 8.
[5]Material on this and pages 149–153 reprinted from National Citizens' Coalition for Nursing Home Reform.

- Arrange (perhaps through library club volunteers) for transportation for residents to visit the library for individual pleasure, to participate in group activities, to volunteer, etc.
- Provide information regarding long-term care to the community, including films, books, copies of directories or brochures with information about facilities, copies of state inspection reports, legislative and regulatory reports, etc.

Mental Health Centers and Other Mental Health Services

- Provide specialists to work directly with individual nursing home residents and groups of residents, including follow-up services to persons "deinstitutionalized" from mental institutions.
- Work with and train nursing home staff and other health professionals dealing with the institutionalized elderly.
- Assist with issues, situations relating to incompetency, guardianship and other protective actions.

Special Interest Organizations and Clubs

- Community Environmental Council can provide services. (In Washington State, one nursing home advocate convinced the Spokane Environmental Council that it should spend time advocating for reform of "the last environment for many of the community's elderly.")
- Red Cross can provide assistance in developing disaster plans and in training highschool students and others to work with ill and disabled elderly.
- Folklore Society can conduct special shows and events for residents or assist them in attending community events. Experience and history of residents can be utilized in discovering new information and talents.

Social Service Agencies and Organizations

- Vocational Rehabilitation can provide outreach services to nursing home residents to assist them as needed. VR can share information with providers on community rehabilitative services and help provide educational programs for nursing home staff.

- Social services caseworkers can help identify resident and facility needs and help locate community resources to meet those needs.
- Salvation Army Social Services programs can assist nursing home staff in their work with alcoholics.

Park and Recreational Services

- Organize and provide special programs such as a "periodic" swim night; nature walks or films; share routinely developed programs of entertainment with nursing homes either on the grounds of nursing homes where the neighbors can participate or help arrange transportation to events.

Private Community Clubs

- Garden Club can provide flower shows; hold meetings in nursing homes; assist residents in gardening on facility grounds or in the facility.
- Local "Round-up" Club can provide special seating space, help arrange transportation for residents to rodeo events. Small partial "parades" can be taken to facilities to perform for residents.
- Sorority/fraternity clubs can provide friendly visiting services, transportation, research on nursing home issues and needs, etc.
- "Brownies," Girl Scouts, 4-H, and others can provide on-going visiting services (i.e. adopt a grandparent); organize and conduct "oral history" surveys/interviews with residents to help provide the libraries with community historical information.

The Media

- Help generate more resources, interest and information in the community by writing feature stories and presenting special programs on residents and nursing home services and activities; keep community generally informed of nursing home activities, including "the good and the bad."

Funding Organizations

- Help community identify needs through research and community exploration and contacts.
- Provide financial resources for model projects, research and resource development.

Educational Institutions

- High School volunteer services to residents through special courses such as homemaking, agriculture, etc. Informational programs in nursing homes to help keep residents informed.
- Identify residents with special skills and information and make arrangements for this to be shared with students in schools (at all levels). Use nursing home residents as tutors.
- High schools, community junior colleges and universities can generate courses which will motivate and prepare students to work with the elderly. Also arrange for special research by students which will lead to improved life for the elderly in institutions.
- Establish adult education courses in nursing homes so that residents can attend and even receive high school diplomas, if interested.

Public Health Agencies

- Provide information and guidelines for minimal standards of care; monitor services to assure implementation; identify resident and facility needs and help develop resources.
- Provide special training programs for nursing home staff, community groups and agencies.

Medical Care and Other Specialist Health Care

- Provide training programs on geriatrics and institutional care which will motivate health care providers and generate improved services.

- Monitor general health care delivery in community nursing home facilities and work towards improvements needed by identifying problems and needs; assist in holding health professionals accountable through peer group pressure and professional associations.
- Volunteer special services not covered by regular reimbursement programs (i.e. preventive dental and vision care).
- Arrange shared responsibilities to assure adequate medical and health care services to facilities.

Fire and Safety Agencies (Departments)

- Provide monitoring and educational services; assistance with fire drills; assist with development of facility disaster plans and assist in arranging community involvement and acceptance of responsibilities related to disaster plans.

Hospitals and Other Health Care Institutions

- Assist in the development and delivery of training programs directed to present or potential nursing home workers.
- Help monitor nursing home care and identify needs of facilities and residents.
- Arrange for sharing of special rehabilitative equipment and services.
- Develop programs to share doctors, nurses and other health care professionals in training programs.

Businesses and Business Organizations

- Help raise funds, solicit donations for special equipment for facilities, special items for residents (i.e. electric wheelchairs not always covered by reimbursement rates).
- Donate special services, supplies, products, such as

  —car companies provide transportation to special community events

  —clothing stores offer special discount for nursing home residents; organize periodic special shopping days; provide style shows in nursing homes featuring older person's clothing; order special low-cost or speciality items for purchase by facilities or residents (i.e. clothing for the disabled).

—restaurants feature and organize a periodic special discount (or free) luncheon "out" for all residents who can participate. Restaurants could "take turns" so that several opportunities are offered each year. Clubs and special groups can assist by providing transportation and volunteer waitress service.

—Banks provide low-cost or free counseling services on banking, retirement income matters, partly by sending representatives periodically to facilities to be available to residents. Work with facility administration to provide best possible banking service for minimal patient fund accounts.

Citizen Involvement (Individuals, groups, ombudsman programs)

• Assist in identifying resident and facility needs and assist in generating resources to meet those needs.

• Monitor quality of care and advocate for improved services.

• Provide friendly visiting services, advocacy services for residents and assist in working with facility personnel and families to help resolve problems.

• Serve the community by providing public education and by organizing more citizens and groups to get involved.

The best nursing homes are those that recognize their role as a part of the total community and that are located in communities where the services of such institutions are seen to have value and purpose. This means the community at large will need information since most citizens will have little cause to know what a nursing home is and is not.

The best people to put such a network into action are you, the caregiving families. When you start to talk about the values of nursing home care and the need for more and better care to those in the community who have remained uninvolved, good things could begin to happen.

And What about the Future?

The news is positive. Nursing homes themselves are realizing the importance of reaching out to the community. Innovative programming is becoming more commonplace than ever before. In one nursing home, the food service instituted a Sunday dinner program for seniors in the community. People who attended the program did not necessarily have a relative in the home. They just lived in the neighborhood. By coming to the home for Sunday dinner, they began to accept the institution as a viable part of the community rather than a place to be avoided at all costs.

In another home, activity directors organized an AA (Alcoholics Anonymous) group for residents and staff. The result was more than the usual support such a group gives recovering alcoholics. It included the added benefit of having staff and residents interact as equals with the result that they became more connected in their daily contact with one another.

Many homes are opening adult daycare centers, providing a continuum of care to serve those who are frail but can still live at home to those who need more constant care through residency in the nursing home.

The entire idea of a family council is relatively new as of this writing. Resident councils were mandated by several states years ago, but the concept of the family council has only just begun to be developed. A national organization has sprung up to help in the coordination of efforts to organize more family and resident councils. The group is National Coalition of Resident Councils for Nursing Home Residents, 3231 First Avenue, S., Minneapolis, MN 55408.

And while progress is far too slow, strides are being made toward caring for the whole person. One of the provisions of the nursing home reform act of 1987 is that any home with over 120 beds must have on staff a social worker and "professionally trained" activity coordinators. Are you surprised that such a mandate was necessary? Don't be. It is but one example of the kind of vigilance and concern for quality that is needed.

For too long the total concentration has been on providing minimal physical and custodial care for residents, especially those residents whose pay source was Medicaid. And this is not the fault of the nursing home industry alone. Some advocacy is finally underway to see that *basic* care includes such "luxuries" as counseling and mental health care, ancillary medical services such as dental, foot, and eye care, and rehabilitative therapies.

A Final Word

Nursing homes have been and will continue to be a vital link in the continuum of long-term care available to the citizens of this country. People coming to nursing homes today are more frail and much sicker than they have been in the past. But the reason for this turn of events is positive—Americans are able to maintain themselves at home with the help of caregivers and community assistance well into their later years. And do not forget that 80 percent of all persons in the United States never need nursing home care at all.

In many ways, these are pioneering times for long-term care. Never before have there been so many people living for so long. Never before have there been the need for and development of so many alternative programs for services. Never before have caregivers been called upon to serve for such long periods. Never before have there been so many choices. And never before has the nursing home been faced with such a need to grow and develop and connect with the community it serves. You, as a caregiver and member of the nursing home team, are an essential part of that growth and development.

Appendix A

State Long-Term Care Ombudsperson Offices

ALABAMA
COMMISSION ON AGING
502 Washington Avenue
Montgomery, AL 36130
(205) 261-5643

ALASKA
OLDER ALASKANS
  OMBUDSMAN
2600 Denali Street, Suite 303
Anchorage, AK 99503-2740
(907) 279-2232

ARIZONA
AGING & ADULT
  ADMINISTRATION
1400 W. Washington Street
P.O. Box 6123
Phoenix, AZ 85007
(602) 255-4446

ARKANSAS
OFFICE ON AGING AND
  ADULT SERVICES
Department of Human Services
Suite 1428, Donaghey Building
7th and Main Streets
Little Rock, AR 72201
(501) 371-2441

CALIFORNIA
CALIFORNIA DEPARTMENT
  ON AGING
1020 19th Street
Sacramento, CA 95814
(916) 323-6681

COLORADO
MEDICAL CARE &
  RESEARCH FOUNDATION
1565 Clarkson Street
Denver, CO 80218
(303) 830-7744

CONNECTICUT
CONNECTICUT
  DEPARTMENT ON AGING
175 Main Street
Hartford, CT 06106
(203) 566-7770

DELAWARE
DIVISION ON AGING
Milford State Service Center
11–13 Church Avenue
Milford, DE 19963
(302) 422-1386

SOURCE: Nursing Home Life: A Guide for Residents and Families (Washington,
D.C.: American Association of Retired Persons, 1987).

156

DISTRICT OF COLUMBIA
LEGAL COUNSEL FOR
  THE ELDERLY
1331 H Street, NW
Washington, DC 20005
(202) 662-4933

FLORIDA
STATE LONG TERM CARE
  OMBUDSMAN COMMITTEE
Department of Health and
  Rehabilitative Services
Building 1, #308
1317 Winewood Boulevard
Tallahassee, FL 32301
(904) 488-6190

GEORGIA
OFFICE OF AGING
Department of Human Resources
Room 632
878 Peachtree Street, N.E.
Atlanta, GA 30389
(404) 894-5833

HAWAII
HAWAII EXECUTIVE OFFICE
  ON AGING
335 Merchant Street, Room 241
Honolulu, HI 96813
(808) 548-2593

IDAHO
IDAHO OFFICE ON AGING
State House, Room 114
Boise, ID 83720
(208) 334-3833

ILLINOIS
DEPARTMENT ON AGING
421 East Capitol Avenue
Springfield, IL 62701
(217) 785-5186

INDIANA
INDIANA DEPARTMENT OF
  AGING AND ADULT
  COMMUNITY SERVICES
Capitol Center, 251 North Illinois
Indianapolis, IN 46207-7083
(317) 232-7115

IOWA
COMMISSION ON THE AGING
Jewett Building, Suite 236
916 Grand Avenue
Des Moines, IA 50319
(515) 281-5187

KANSAS
DEPARTMENT ON AGING
610 West Tenth Street
Topeka, KS 66612
(913) 296-4986

KENTUCKY
DIVISION FOR AGING
  SERVICES
Department of Human Resources
275 East Main Street
Frankfort, KY 40601
(501) 564-6930

LOUISIANA
GOVERNOR'S OFFICE OF
  ELDERLY AFFAIRS
4528 Bennington Avenue
P.O. Box 80374
Baton Rouge, LA 70898-3074
(504) 925-1700

MAINE
MAINE COMMITTEE
  ON AGING
Station 11, State House
Augusta, ME 04333
(207) 289-3658

MARYLAND
MARYLAND OFFICE ON
 AGING
301 West Preston Street
Baltimore, MD 21201
(301) 225-1100

MASSACHUSETTS
MASSACHUSETTS
 EXECUTIVE OFFICE OF
 ELDER AFFAIRS
38 Chauncy Street
Boston, MA 02111
(617) 727-7273

MICHIGAN
CITIZENS FOR BETTER CARE
1627 East Kalamazoo
Lansing, MI 48917
(517) 482-1297

MINNESOTA
MINNESOTA BOARD ON
 AGING
Metro Square Building, Room 204
7th and Robert Streets
St. Paul, MN 55101
(612) 296-7465

MISSISSIPPI
MISSISSIPPI COUNCIL ON
 AGING
301 West Pearl Street
Jackson, MS 39203-3092
(601) 949-2013

MISSOURI
DIVISION ON AGING
Department of Social Services
P.O. Box 1337
505 Missouri Boulevard
Jefferson City, MO 65102
(314) 751-3082

MONTANA
SENIORS' OFFICE OF
 LEGAL AND OMBUDSMAN
 SERVICES
P.O. Box 232, Capitol Station
Helena, MT 59620
(406) 444-4204

NEBRASKA
DEPARTMENT ON AGING
P.O. Box 95044
301 Centennial Mall-South
Lincoln, NE 68509
(402) 471-2307

NEVADA
DIVISION OF AGING
 SERVICES
Department of Human Resources
Kinkead Building, Room 101
505 East King Street
Carson City, NV 89710
(702) 885-4210

NEW HAMPSHIRE
NEW HAMPSHIRE STATE
 COUNCIL ON AGING
Prescott Park
105 Loudon Road, Building #3
Concord, NH 03301
(603) 271-2751

NEW JERSEY
OFFICE OF THE
 OMBUDSMAN FOR THE
 INSTITUTIONALIZED
 ELDERLY
Room 305, CN808
28 West State Street
Trenton, NJ 08625-0807
(609) 292-8016

NEW MEXICO
STATE AGENCY ON AGING
LaVilla Rivera Building, 4th Floor
224 East Palace Avenue
Santa Fe, NM 87501
(505) 827-7640

NEW YORK
OFFICE FOR THE AGING
Agency Building #2
Empire State Plaza
Albany, NY 12223
(518) 474-0108

NORTH CAROLINA
NORTH CAROLINA
  DEPARTMENT OF
  HUMAN RESOURCES
Division of Aging
Kirby Building
1985 Umpstead Drive
Raleigh, NC 27603
(919) 733-3983

NORTH DAKOTA
AGING SERVICES DIVISION
Department of Human Services
State Capitol Building
Bismarck, ND 58505
(701) 224-2577

OHIO
OHIO DEPARTMENT ON
  AGING
50 W. Broad Street, 9th Floor
Columbus, OH 43215
(614) 466-9927

OKLAHOMA
SPECIAL UNIT ON AGING
Department of Human Services
P.O. Box 25352
Oklahoma City, OK 73125
(405) 521-2281

OREGON
OFFICE OF LONG TERM
  CARE OMBUDSMAN
2475 Lancaster Drive
Building B, #9
Salem, OR 97310
(503) 378-6533

PENNSYLVANIA
DEPARTMENT OF AGING
Barto Building
231 State Street
Harrisburg, PA 17101
(717) 783-7247

PUERTO RICO
GERICULTURE COMMISSION
Department of Social Services
G.P.O. Box 11398
Santurce, PR 00910
(809) 722-2429

RHODE ISLAND
RHODE ISLAND
  DEPARTMENT OF
  ELDERLY AFFAIRS
79 Washington Street
Providence, RI 02903
(401) 277-6880

SOUTH CAROLINA
OFFICE OF THE GOVERNOR
  DIVISION OF OMBUDSMAN
  AND CITIZENS' SERVICES
1205 Pendleton Street
Columbia, SC 29201
(803) 734-0457

SOUTH DAKOTA
OFFICE OF ADULT SERVICES
  AND AGING
Department of Social Services
Richard F. Kneip Building
700 N. Illinois Street
Pierre, SD 57501-2291
(605) 773-3656

TENNESSEE
COMMISSION ON AGING
715 Tennessee Building
535 Church Street
Nashville, TN 37219
(615) 741-2056

TEXAS
TEXAS DEPARTMENT ON
  AGING
P.O. Box 12786 Capitol Station
Austin, TX 78704
(512) 444-2727

UTAH
DIVISION OF AGING & ADULT
  SERVICES
Department of Social Services
150 W. North Temple, Room 4A
Salt Lake City, UT 04103
(801) 533-6422

VERMONT
VERMONT OFFICE ON AGING
103 South Main Street
Waterbury, VT 05676
(802) 241-2400

VIRGINIA
DEPARTMENT FOR THE
  AGING
101 N. 14th Street, 18th Floor
James Monroe Building
Richmond, Virginia 23219
(804) 225-2912

WASHINGTON
DIVISION OF AUDIT
Department of Social & Health
  Services
MS OB-44-Y
Olympia, WA 98504
(206) 586-2258

WEST VIRGINIA
COMMISSION ON AGING
State Capitol Complex
Charleston, WV 25305
(304) 348-3317

WISCONSIN
BOARD ON AGING AND
  LONG TERM CARE
819 North 6th, Room 619
Milwaukee, WI 53203-1664
(414) 227-4386

WYOMING
WYOMING STATE BAR
  ASSOCIATION
900 8th Street
Wheatland, WY 82201
(307) 322-5553

Appendix B

Resident Rights

The following nursing home reform amendments affecting residents' rights were enacted by Congress as a part of the Omnibus Budget Reconciliation Act in December 1987. The new law will be administered by the Department of Health and Human Services and mandates that any home participating in Medicare or Medicaid programs ensure the following rights to residents.

1. The new law places a federal emphasis on the importance of quality of life (not just quality of care) for each resident. This provision is designed to ensure rights to dignity, choice, and autonomy.
2. Nursing homes are required to provide services and activities designed to "attain or maintain the highest practicable physical, mental, and psychosocial well-being of each resident in accordance with a written plan of care." The law further states that this care plan is to be prepared with every possible participation by the resident or the resident's family or guardian.
3. Residents have the right to participate in administration of the facility's programs through their right to assemble and act through a resident's council and as individuals.
4. The law protects specific individual rights for every resident including:
   • the right to choose a personal physician
   • the right to full information in advance and opportunity to participate in planning and making any changes in their care and treatment plans

- the right to voice grievances without discrimination or reprisal as well as the right to receive prompt response to those grievances
- the right to organize and participate in resident (and family) advocacy groups
- the right to choose and participate in social, religious, and community activities
- the right to privacy for medical treatments, personal visits, written and telephone communications, and meetings with others of their choice
- the right to confidentiality of personal and clinical records
- the right to be free of physical or chemical restraints used for convenience of the staff
- the right to freedom from abuse (physical or mental), punishment, or restraint for disciplinary reasons
- the right to have restraints (either chemical or physical) used only under the express written direction of the resident's physician as part of the care plan for a specific condition and with annual review of appropriateness.

5. Residents also have the right to certain basic information including:
   - access to the home's latest inspection results
   - notification of any plan to change room or roommate
   - information in writing about rights and procedures for filing grievances
   - written information about costs and charges for basic and extra services
   - written information on applying for benefits under Title XIX of Medicaid

6. The new laws mandate that facilities must guarantee certain rights pertaining to visitors and transfers including:
   - the right to immediate access to the resident by his or her personal physician, the health department, or the ombudsperson
   - the right to immediate visits (meaning at any time, not just during stated visiting hours) by the resident's family at the resident's request

• the right of the resident to choose to accept visits by organizations or individuals providing services from outside the home (such as legal, health, or social services)

• the right to remain in the facility without fear of transfer or discharge unless transfer is necessary in order for resident to receive public funding, transfer or discharge is necessary because the current level of care is inappropriate (as in the case where a resident improves to such a degree that a skilled level of care is no longer necessary), transfer or discharge is necessary because resident is a danger to the health or safety of other residents, or transfer or discharge is necessary because the resident fails to pay for services provided at his or her request

[Regarding transfer, the new law states that residents are to receive 30 days notice if possible or as much advance notice as possible when health conditions require a more immediate transfer. The resident has the right to appeal the decision to transfer and the right to request the bed be held in the event the transfer is temporary (as to a hospital). If the temporary stay lasts longer than the allowable days for holding a bed, the resident has the right to request the next available bed.]

7. Protections for the personal funds of nursing home residents are also covered in the new federal reforms. The nursing home cannot require a resident to deposit personal funds to the facility, but if the resident chooses to do so, the facility must:

• keep funds over $50 in an interest-bearing account that is separate from the facility's account

• keep other funds available through a petty cash fund

• keep complete and accurate accounts with written records of all transactions that are available for review by the resident or his or her representative

• notify Title XIX (Medicaid) residents when their account balance reaches limits that will affect eligibility

• turn funds over to resident's trustee upon the death of the resident

• not charge residents paying under Title XIX for any item or service already covered by Medicaid funds

8. Finally, residents who are eligible to receive care under Title XIX funds of the Medicaid program are protected under this federal law from:

   • discrimination in terms of transfers, discharge, and provision of services

   • requirements to waive rights to Medicaid coverage in order to satisfy certain residency requirements

   • requirements for third-party payments as a condition of admission to or continued stay in the facility

   • solicitations for gifts, donations, or "other consideration" as a precondition for continued residency

Appendix C

Omnibus Reconciliation Budget Act of 1987 Nursing Home Reforms

In addition to guarantees of certain rights for residents of nursing homes, the new federal nursing home reforms include the following measures to be phased in over a two-year period:

Effective in 1988—

• establish national standards for training of nurses' aides

• identification of Medicaid-covered services by individual states with federal regulation regarding those services in place

• development of standards and criteria for monitoring nurse staffing requirements

Effective in 1989—

• set guidelines for appeals process for resident transfers
• approve nurses' aide training standards
• implement standards for nursing home administrators in each state
• establish a nurses' aide registry in each state

Effective in 1990—

• develop a national standard for surveys
• develop a national standard for assessing residents
• begin aide training and review program
• eliminate distinction between intermediate and skilled care facilities

[The reform act is designed to become fully effective by October 1, 1990.]

For Further Reading

American Association of Retired Persons. *Nursing Home Life: A Guide for Residents and Families.* Washington, DC: AARP, 1987.

Bennett, Clifford. *Nursing Home Life: What It Is and What It Could Be.* New York: The Tiresias Press, 1980.

Fox, Nancy. *You, Your Parent, and the Nursing Home: The Family's Guide to Long Term Care.* Buffalo: Prometheus Books, 1986.

Hunter, Laura Russell. *The Rest of My Life.* Stanford, CT: Growing Pains Press, 1981.

Sollenberger, Opal Hutchins. *I Chose to Live in a Nursing Home.* Elgin, IL: David C. Cook Publishing Co., 1980.

U.S. Department of Health and Human Services. *How to Select a Nursing Home.* Washington, DC: Government Printing Office, 1980.

Index

167

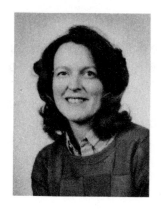

About the Author

Jo Horne has spent much of her adult life working with organizations caring for the aging. She is also a writer and the author of the AARP Book *Caregiving: Helping an Aging Loved One* and coauthor with Leo Baldwin of *Homesharing and Other Lifestyle Options*. Her interest in both subjects comes from the clients and families who come to the adult daycare center in Milwaukee where she is an administrator with her husband, Larry Schmidt.

Horne has a master's degree in communication from the University of Cincinnati. She has completed the Intensive Training Program of the Midwest Geriatric Education Center and was named a Fellow in 1988. The center—which is a major link in a nationwide network of regional education centers and is funded by the U.S. Department of Health and Human Services—accepts a limited number of geriatric professionals as students who will use what they learn to educate other professionals and service providers. Horne was accepted in response to her wish to continue educating others through her writing. Following her completion of the intensive training program, Horne was awarded a grant by the Association of University Programs in Health Administration (AUPHA) to develop a curriculum module on the topic of Long-Term Care—Continuum of Care.

Since *Caregiving* was published, Horne has appeared on national television and radio talk shows and has spoken to many groups on issues related to caregiving and aging. She is a member of the Gerontological Society of America, the Older Women's League, the National Council on the Aging, and the Alzheimer's Disease and Related Disorders Association.

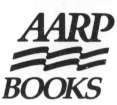
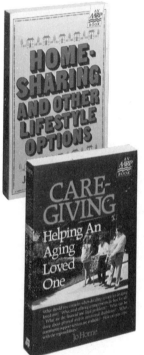
8652